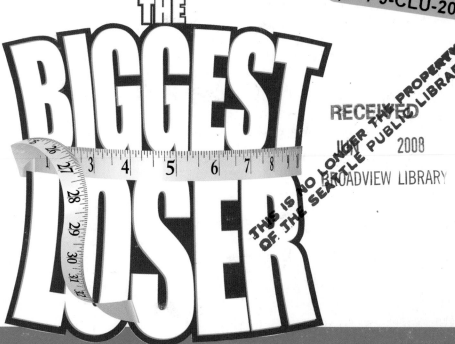

THE BIGGEST LOSER

SUCCESS SECRETS

The Wisdom, Motivation, and Inspiration to Lose Weight—and Keep It Off!

The Biggest Loser Experts and Cast
with Maggie Greenwood-Robinson, PhD

Library of Congress Cataloging-in-Publication Data

The Biggest Loser success secrets : the wisdom, motivation, and inspiration to lose weight and keep it off! / The Biggest Loser experts and cast with Maggie Greenwood-Robinson.
    p.   cm.
Includes bibliographical references and index.
ISBN-13 978–1–59486–799–6   paperback
ISBN-10 1–59486–799–2   paperback
1. Physical fitness.   2. Weight loss.   I. Greenwood-Robinson, Maggie.   II. Biggest loser (Television program).
RA781.B487 2008
613.7—dc22   2008000076

Distributed to the trade by Macmillan

2   4   6   8   10   9   7   5   3   1   paperback

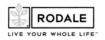

We inspire and enable people to improve their lives and the world around them

For more of our products visit **rodalestore.com** or call 800-848-4735

Product Development & Direction:

Chad Bennett, Dave Broome, Cindy Chang, Neysa Gordon, Mark Koops, Kim Niemi

NBCU, Reveille, 25/7 Productions and 3Ball Productions would like to thank the many people who gave their time and energy to this project:

Jenna Alifante, Stephen Andrade, Dana Arnett, Sebastian Attie, Matt Assmus, Nancy N. Bailey, Beth Bazar, Maria Bohe, Dave Broome, Jen Busch, *The Biggest Loser* contestants, Jill Carmen, Cindy Chang, Scot Chastain, Ben Cohen, Marie Connolly, Mary Conte, Jason Cooper, Dan Curran, Dr. Michael Dansinger, Camilla Dhanak, Cori Diamond, Hayley Dickson, Milissa Douponce, Leslie Duong, Nancy Elgin, Jenny Ellis, Kat Elmore, John Farrell, Cheryl Forberg, Kurt Ford, Wendy Gable, Jeff Gaspin, Christina Gaugler, Marc Graboff, Maggie Greenwood-Robinson, Erica Gruen, Heather Halloway, Nancy Hancock, Libby Hansen, Bob Harper, Shelli Hill, Dr. Robert Huizenga, Helen Jorda, Allison Kaz, Connie Kempany, Dr. Jennifer Kerns, Jessica Kirby, Loretta Kraft, Chris Krogermeier, Laura Kuhn, Beth Lamb, Jessica Lane, Melissa Leffler, Todd Lubin, Roni Lubliner, Alan Lundgren, Kim Lyons, Carole MacDonal, Vince Manze, Rebecca Marks, Joaquin Mesa, Jillian Michaels, Lily Milkovic-Jakal, John Miller, Ann Morteo, Kam Naderi, Todd Nelson, Bill Ostroff, Carole Panick, Joanne Park, Trae Patton, Liz Perl, Jerry Petry, Craig Plestis, Chris Rhoads, Lee Rierson, Melissa Roberson, Beth Roberts, J. D. Roth, Jessica Roth, Jennifer Scott, Robin Shallow, Ben Silverman, Carrie Simons, Hayley Sneiderman, Mitch Steele, Lee Straus, Amy Super, Kelia Tardiff, Deborah Thomas, Stacey Ward, Liza Whitcraft, Julie Will, Bob Wright, Yong Yam, Jeff Zucker

Contents

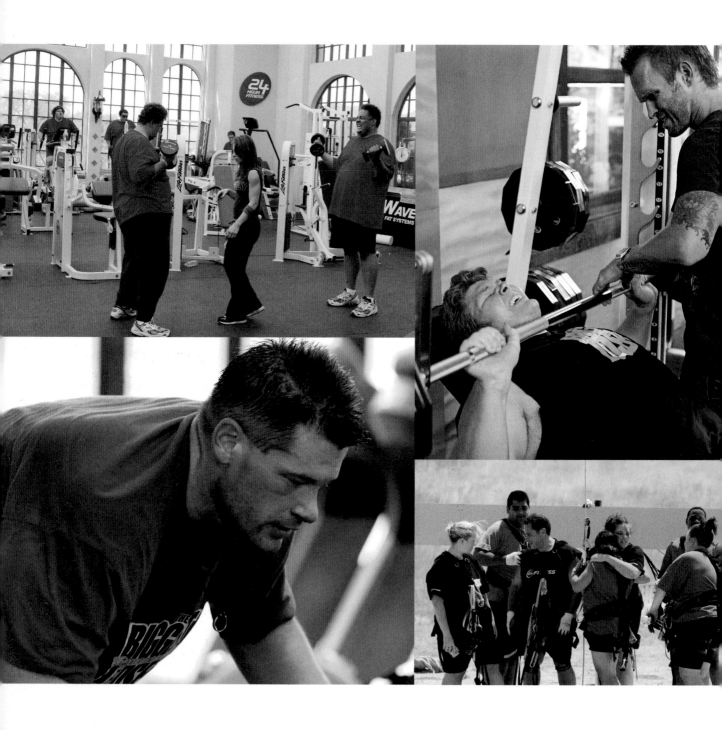

Introduction

The Biggest Loser Secrets and Strategies . . . Revealed!

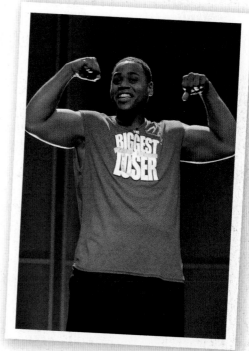

What if you had the power to create the body you never dreamed was possible? What if you started getting in such great shape that you felt attractive and joyful and in control of your life? What if you experienced a total transformation that allowed you to be all you can be? What if you felt you could live like this—healthy, active, and full of vibrancy—for the rest of your life?

I know these claims sound outlandish, but they're within your grasp—in fact, the power to change is right in your hands! This book has the answers you've been searching for. It doesn't matter whether you're a devoted fan of NBC's hit weight-loss show *The Biggest Loser* or have never even heard of it—this book will show you how to create the body you want and change your health and fitness destiny dramatically and permanently.

Now in its fifth season, *The Biggest Loser* has featured contestants who weighed more than 200, 300, or 400 pounds when they started and then went on to achieve their goal weights in astonishing flab-to-fab transformations. Many of them have kept their weight off successfully, a feat that is virtually unheard of in today's heavyweight society.

If you watch the show, you know the contestants' physical and mental limits are tested during grueling challenges, and you've seen them dealing with the week-to-week threat of being ousted by their teammates if they're weighing the group down. What you don't see is what happens during the rest of the week on campus—the meals of healthy, low-fat protein and high-nutrient vegetables and fruits; the calorie monitoring; the hours of exercising; and the advice and support from a team of experts, all working toward the same goal: to help the cast members lose weight now, keep it off later, and restore their hope for living happy and healthy lives. But even with a team of experts, when it comes to losing weight permanently, no one can do it for the contestants but themselves.

So, how do they do it?

This book takes you behind the scenes of the show to give you the real-life scoop from the contestants on how they achieved such astonishing transformations. Additionally, you'll get to revisit many of your favorite contestants from past seasons who have been successful at the most difficult part of weight loss—keeping it off.

If you have ever tried to lose weight on your own, you know how tough it is. It's easy to get discouraged when you don't drop pounds, and you start to think that losing weight is an impossible dream. The next thing you know, you start cheating. A little treat here, a reward there, and pretty soon you've thrown in the towel. Clearly, staying motivated is the keystone of success when you are working to lose weight and keep it off. As anyone who's watched the show knows, *The Biggest Loser* has given millions of people hope and inspiration to lose weight and keep it off, and this book will do the same. In just three and a half short years, *The Biggest Loser* has become a worldwide phenomenon. Now airing in 90 countries with original shows produced in 25, this is a weight-loss program that is changing lives on a global scale. In addition to the television show, *The Biggest Loser* program has created a best-selling series of diet and fitness books, a best-selling workout DVD, and of course, a huge, supportive online community with more than 300,000 members. But most important, it has helped hundreds of thousands of people realize their dreams and begin living the lives they were meant to live. You can, too.

By way of introduction, here are the contestants who will help you achieve your goals.

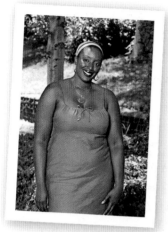

Andrea "Drea" Baptiste

Before: 215 pounds

After: 156 pounds

As an athlete in high school and college and then as a personal trainer with a degree in exercise physiology, Drea had to stay in top form. But when she became focused on her new career as a pharmaceutical sales rep, exercising and eating healthy meals became less of a priority. She indulged in junk food and rarely worked out, making up every excuse in the book not to go to the gym. Before long, she was popping out of size 16 clothes. When she finally stepped on the scale, the needle stuck at 215 pounds. She knew she couldn't sit back and do nothing.

During her *Biggest Loser* experience, she shed 59 pounds, and she's kept it off. "Losing this weight has been by far the most rewarding opportunity of my life," she says. "I don't see anything that could possibly beat this in my past, and I don't foresee anything possibly coming close to this in my future, because this experience has been a complete change, inside and out."

The combination of prime-time exposure and dramatic weight loss helped Drea realize a long-delayed dream. Recently, she opened her own personal-training and life-coaching center, which offers lifestyle and weight-management guidance.

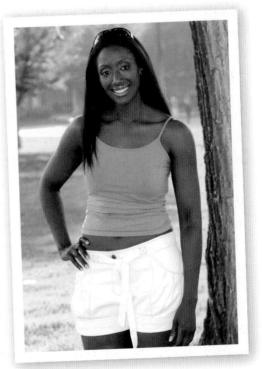

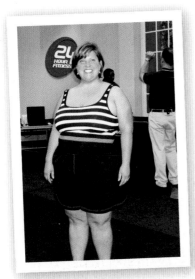

Kelly MacFarland

Before: 223 pounds

After: 151 pounds

Kelly has many roles in life: an employee by day, a stand-up comic at night, and a food addict all the time. "My friends and I would always go out to dinner, always have drinks, and always indulge in everything."

As a child, Kelly dreamed of being a dancer on Broadway. Those dreams were dashed as she started filling out all over and got bigger than most other girls her age. "I started feeling self-conscious about my body. I would get small, then I would get big again, and then small again and big. This last time, I just got big and stayed that way."

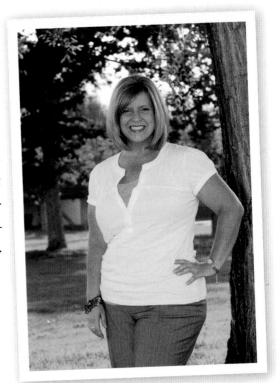

At 223 pounds, the 34-year-old comedian had become so heavy that her stand-up act turned into a fat joke. Yet all of that weight on her 5-foot frame was no laughing matter. Once she became a contestant on *The Biggest Loser*, she lost 72 pounds—and best of all, she has kept 65 of those pounds off. Kelly appeared on *The Biggest Loser* reunion special in 2007, looking fit and fabulous. "I consider being on *The Biggest Loser* a monumental experience. I'm a different person, and I like me."

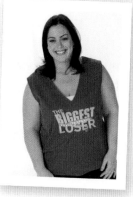

Andrea Overstreet

Before: 220 pounds
After: 145 pounds

Unlike many other contestants, Andrea did not always have a weight problem—in fact, she was athletic and fit for most of her life. But when she was pregnant with her daughter, she gained 100 pounds. "I lost some, but then regained it and more," she says. "I've always played sports—soccer, softball, and, most recently, hockey—but I stopped when the gear didn't fit and I couldn't move. It just wasn't fun."

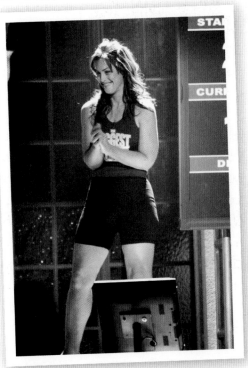

Andrea kept piling on the pounds and struggled to take them back off. Not surprisingly, she wanted to regain the strong, beautiful body she once had. *The Biggest Loser* kicked her into action, and once she got moving there was no stopping her. Andrea always had a vision of herself as a princess; now she looks and feels like one, too—even a couple of years after her phenomenal experience on *The Biggest Loser*. "How do I possibly put it into words? It was downright amazing. It was a once-in-a-lifetime chance that I am very fortunate to have been given."

Andrea now has her own Web site, where she shares a number of the healthy lifestyle tips she uses to maintain her great shape.

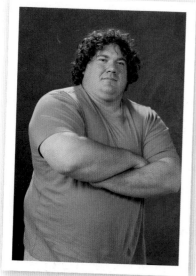

Matt Hoover: Winner, Season 2

Before: 339 pounds

After: 182 pounds

Matt was the NCAA Iowa State Champion in wrestling, and he was bound for the Olympics—until an injury stopped him in his tracks. After that, he gained so much weight that reentering competitive sports seemed like an impossible dream. But he never lost the will to win, and that is precisely what he did. After dropping an amazing 157 pounds, he was crowned the Biggest Loser in Season 2. Matt has achieved his goal of "being an athlete again," and he also found love: He and fellow cast member Suzy Preston got married, and Suzy recently gave birth to their son, Rex. Like many new parents, Matt and Suzy have gained back some weight since Rex's arrival—but they are confident they will return to their svelte figures, thanks to the maintenance skills they learned on *The Biggest Loser*.

Matt is now a full-time motivational speaker. He also works with developmentally challenged and autistic children. Since winning the Season 2 title, he has gained back some weight, but has managed to keep off 100 pounds—an inspiring, commendable feat. Matt has stopped seeing himself as fat—a change in mind-set that has been crucial to his success. "Let yourself be the 'new you,' and you will keep your weight off," he advises.

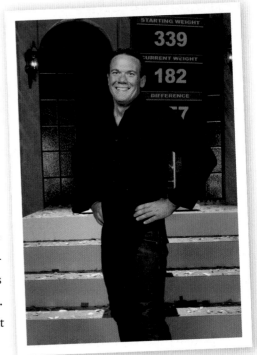

Pete Thomas

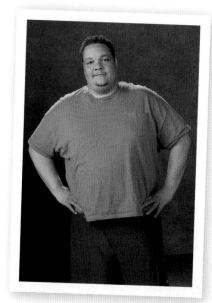

Before: 401 pounds
After: 216 pounds

Pete's weight-gain story is all too common. He fell in love, got married—and got heavy. "After I got married, I gained about 10 pounds a year. I used to play basketball recreationally, about four or five times a week. I stopped playing basketball to spend more time with her and eventually became a couch potato. I've struggled with my weight ever since."

Pete was overweight for simple reasons: He loved to eat (food was his "friend") and didn't exercise. But this devoted husband, whose friends and family considered him the life of the party, knew the time had come to make a change.

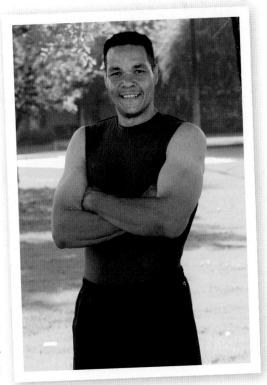

At 401 pounds, Pete knew his health was in serious jeopardy, not least from the dangerously high blood pressure he'd developed. He dug deep and found the determination and drive to lose an astounding 185 pounds. Today, Pete has his own organization, Winning Man (www.winningman.com), through which he coaches and guides others by giving speeches at churches and community group meetings.

If you caught *The Biggest Loser* reunion special in 2007, you saw Pete Thomas bound onto the stage, sporting the same trim, muscular physique that won him Season 2's $100,000 consolation prize. He lost a whopping 185 pounds for the Season 2 finale and has mastered the ability to keep off 165 pounds of it. You'll learn his secrets here.

Suzy Preston: Finalist, Season 2

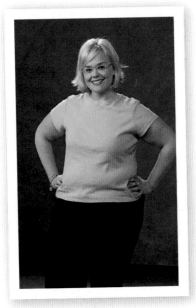

Before: 227 pounds
After: 132 pounds

Suzy spent her high school and young adult years tipping the scales at around 250 pounds. "When I was riding in a car with someone, I'd worry, 'Is my waist spilling over the seat belt?,'" she says. "Was I invading another person's seat on the plane? My weight was always looming in the background."

As a hairdresser, she concentrated her energy on making others feel good and often forgot to focus on herself. But that's what she had to do at the ranch in order to attain her goals of losing weight, feeling confident, and finding the man of her dreams. Little did she know that all of that would actually happen on *The Biggest Loser*. She lost 95 pounds, got in awesome shape, and became the season's second runner-up—and she also discovered true love with Matt Hoover, the winner of Season 2, who is now her husband. She's gained a little weight since giving birth to their son, Rex, but she continues her Biggest Loser lifestyle by watching her diet, exercising daily, and avoiding trigger foods. Suzy says she's now able to be a better person because she takes better care of herself. "I want people to know that they can do this, and they'll come to value themselves in the process."

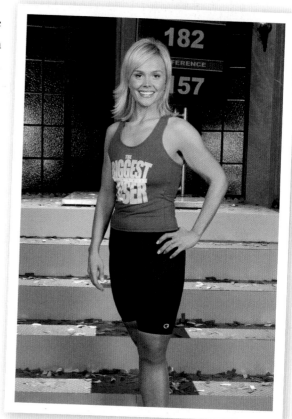

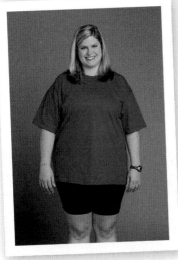

Amy Hildreth

Before: 260 pounds

After: 154 pounds

Blonde, beautiful, and smart, Amy has struggled with her weight since she was a child, but she finally put her foot down. With her fiery personality and confidence, she was able to jettison pizza, fatty foods, and soda in exchange for a healthy lifestyle that enabled her to realize her dreams.

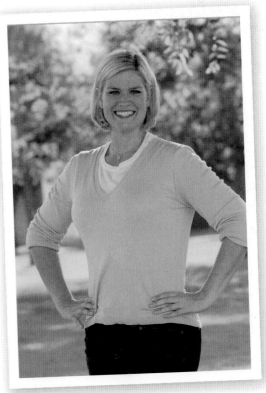

Amy says she began to conquer her weight when she let go of her fear of pushing herself physically. "Bob (Harper's) goal was to get me running," she says. "One day we were running to the gate and back. I felt so exhausted I couldn't move. Bob asked me, 'What are you afraid of?' And he was right, I *could* keep running; I just needed someone to tell me it was okay to push myself."

As a result of being on *The Biggest Loser*, Amy not only learned about eating healthfully, she also fell in love with fellow cast member Marty Wolff. During the 2007 reunion show, Marty proposed to Amy. The couple started their own health business called Reality Wellness, based in Omaha, Nebraska. It's geared toward helping people across the country learn how to become "biggest losers."

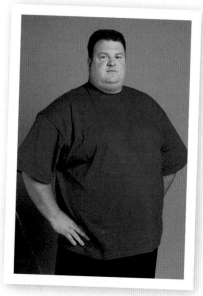

Erik Chopin: Winner, Season 3

Before: 407 pounds
After: 193 pounds

Erik had been an athlete growing up, but after he stopped running twice a day, the weight started piling on. His massive weight gain tremendously impacted his family by limiting the activities he could do with his wife and daughters.

But in Season 3, this Long Island family man and deli owner won the $250,000 prize for his dramatic loss of 214 pounds. He proved to himself—and to America—that you don't necessarily have to undergo gastric bypass surgery (which he was considering) to reverse morbid obesity. Erik also reversed his type 2 diabetes and sleep apnea and brought his elevated blood pressure, cholesterol, and triglyceride levels down to healthy numbers. Although losing the weight was the "hardest thing" he's ever done, Erik smiles today when people call him the Biggest Loser.

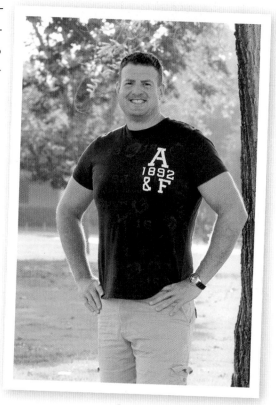

Erik has since sold the deli and tours the country as a motivational speaker. His message: how to lose weight, be successful, and develop a winning attitude. Erik has directed a lot of his efforts toward schools to help stem the epidemic of childhood and teenage obesity. What's more, he has a string of other projects in the works, from a book to an Internet project to a possible television show.

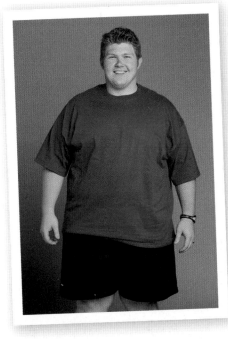

Marty Wolff

Before: 365 pounds

After: 219 pounds

Marty has always taken things to the extreme. As his mother will attest, Marty was described by his doctor at birth as "a big boned boy." And he kept growing. Marty was always one of the biggest kids in his class. As a football player in high school, he was the best. And when Marty sat down for a meal, he would eat and eat . . . and eat.

Marty remembers being called hurtful names and ridiculed throughout his school years. He armored himself with humor and began to believe that being fat was his identity. Soon he found that he was the class clown—likable and popular, no matter what his size. His sense of fun and humor won him a lot of friends.

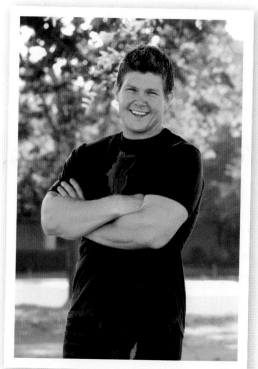

Marty's competitive streak and can-do personality served him well as a *Biggest Loser* contestant: He shed 146 pounds and continues to maintain his loss through healthy eating and regular exercise. Marty knows that maintenance is a lifelong commitment—one that he shares with the love of his life, whom he met at the ranch: fiancée Amy Hildreth. After the show, Marty and Amy were motivated to get their personal training certifications and start helping others lose weight. They created their own company, and together they are taking health and fitness to the rest of America.

Pam Smith

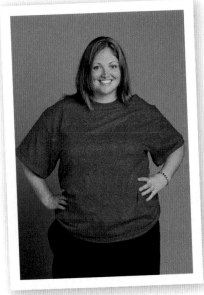

Before: 247 pounds

After: 179 pounds

This Indiana country girl can steal your heart without your ever realizing it. Pam talks a mile a minute, and her charm and personality light up a room. Pam grew up in a simple country home where a trip to the local fast-food joint was considered a family outing, but she doesn't want to pass on the fast-food addiction to her children. And she won't. This devoted wife and mother is staying trim and fit with healthy eating and daily exercise. For her, there's no shame in being called a loser.

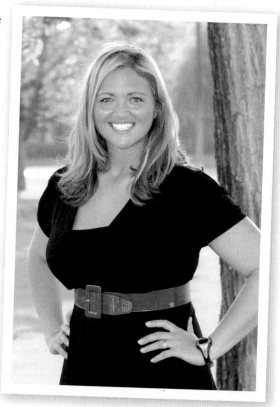

As a fan of the show, Pam was thrilled beyond words to be selected for *The Biggest Loser.* "What's funny, too, is that, at 250 pounds, I didn't think I was fat," she laughs. She calls the experience life changing, but the single hardest thing she's ever done. "I was halfway across the country from my husband and kids for two months."

Pam lost 40 pounds on the ranch before she was eliminated. After she headed home, she lost another 28 pounds and dropped multiple dress sizes. What Pam is really proud of now is that she has kept all but 5 pounds of her weight off. Her simple secret: "Eat well 90 percent of the time."

Pam is now counseling others on how to do the same and has had some impressive success stories of her own. Many of her clients have lost 30, 50, or more pounds.

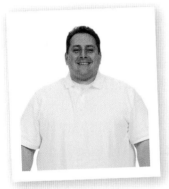

Bill Germanakos: Winner, Season 4

Before: 330 pounds
After: 170 pounds

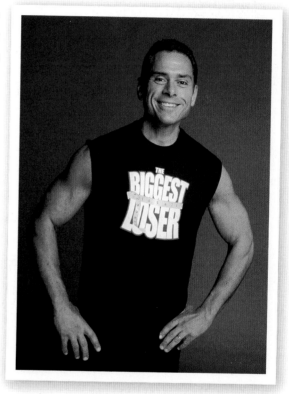

There is a history of heart disease in Bill's family—his father was only 57 years old when he died of a heart attack—so Bill knew he had to start taking responsibility for his own health. Not only did he want to lose weight to live a longer life, he also wanted to be more desirable to his wife, Stephanie. With the help of his brother, Jim, who was also on the show, Bill reached his weight-loss goal. And after reaching it, he was crowned Season 4's Biggest Loser and took home the $250,000 prize. Now he's looking forward to a "whole new life" and plans on staying fit and trim for the rest of it.

He's doing that by using the tools he learned on the ranch. "Honestly, I wish I had known more about the right way to diet and exercise," he says. "As someone who had spent a lot of time on fad diets *and* a lot of time in the gym, I realize now that I really didn't know very much at all."

When he started *The Biggest Loser*, Bill could barely walk up a flight of stairs without stopping to catch his breath, and now he's competing in mini triathlons. "It's a dream come true and something I never even could have imagined. As far as my weight loss goes . . . I still can't believe it. The proof, however, is that I actually fit into my 'goal' pants, which are exactly 10 sizes smaller than the pants I was wearing when the show began."

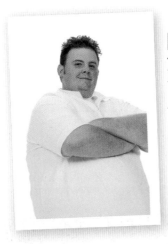

David Griffin

Before: 368 pounds
After: 228 pounds

David is the proud father of four healthy children, and he wants to live a long, fulfilling life as he watches them grow up. David always knew he had a weight problem—he was already obese at 10 years old.

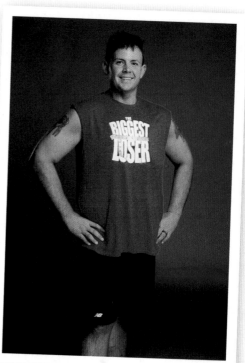

He admits that he was living dangerously. "I didn't have high blood pressure or cholesterol but I was borderline. And that stuff sneaks up on you. Had I gone another year in that shape, who knows what would've happened."

David tried out for the show at the urging of an old friend, a nutritionist. "She knew I needed help," he says. And help it did! After shedding 140 pounds, David says he no longer views food the same way. "I now eat to live, rather than live to eat." He also hopes that his success on the show motivates viewers at home to achieve their goals. "Everyone needs a little inspiration at times. It helps us all to see how much hard work and dedication can change a person's life."

Now, his goal is to be a role model for his children so they never have to suffer the consequences of an unhealthy lifestyle. He has recently been able to return to his favorite activities, like horseback riding and playing basketball and baseball, thanks to his regular exercise program.

Jim Germanakos

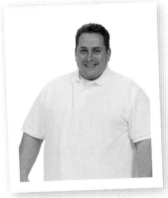

Before: 361 pounds

After: 175 pounds

Jim joined his twin brother, Bill, on a weight-loss journey that changed both of their lives. Jim, like Bill, was rocked by his father's death after a heart attack, and he knew that he had to make big changes in his own life. With the love and support of his wife of 16 years and his three children, Jim got on the right path to a healthier lifestyle and knew that *The Biggest Loser* would help him achieve his ultimate goal of losing weight and becoming fit.

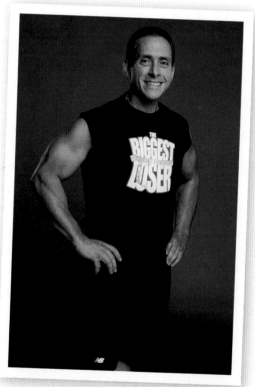

"Like my brother, I had gotten to the point where I was often out of breath, and I realized that being grossly overweight, and a smoker, I could die at any moment," he recalls. "I'm so thankful that I got on the show."

Jim was voted off the show after 5 weeks, but he continued losing weight at home. By the Season 4 finale, he had lost 186 pounds (130 of it at home). Jim won $100,000 for his remarkable success.

"My life has changed for good, forever," he says. "It's a new, healthier way of life now. And I've included my family in my training. I go running and bike riding with my wife. At 41 years old, I feel at least as good as I did when I was 21. I'm a happier person now, definitely."

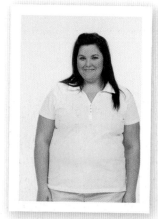

Hollie Self: Finalist, Season 4

Before: 255 pounds
After: 150 pounds

Hollie is a high school English teacher who also works as a cheerleading coach. But her out-of-shape physique made it hard to keep up with the young girls she teaches to cheer. Hollie wasn't happy with her extra weight and knew it was time to make a change. "At some point, you have to take a second and think about what you want your life to be. I decided that I wanted to be healthier, and though it's a long road, so far the rewards far outweigh the struggle," she says.

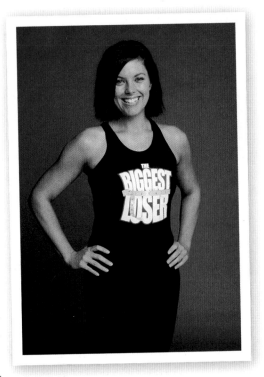

Hollie admits that her months on *The Biggest Loser* were tough. "Watching it from my couch was pretty easy. I thought to myself, 'No problem! I can totally do that!' When you get there and actually start exercising, it is pretty overwhelming."

It may have been tough, but Hollie lost an astonishing 105 pounds and became one of Season 4's finalists. "I have committed to changing my lifestyle," she says. "I know that if I go back to living my life the way I used to, the weight will inevitably come back on."

Hollie has moved to Los Angeles to keep up her healthy new lifestyle and is a trim, positive role model for her students and her cheerleaders.

Isabeau Miller: Finalist, Season 4

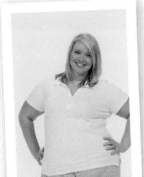

Before: 298 pounds
After: 185 pounds

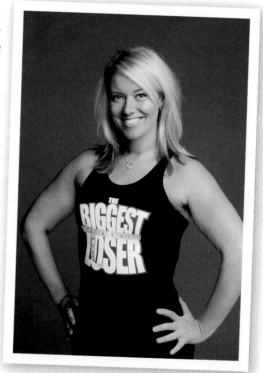

Isabeau used to gorge herself with food, which had essentially become anesthesia for the parts of her life she didn't want to deal with. "Once I had a particularly greasy meal—lots of cheese, sauce, spicy stuff—and it made me feel sick. I remember lying on the bathroom floor and wondering if I was having a heart attack. At 21, that shouldn't even be a question in someone's mind. That's when I knew I had to change."

Isabeau has always dreamed of being a professional singer; she's been writing and performing songs for as long as she can remember. She even took her passion for singing to the ultimate level by graduating from the prestigious Berklee College of Music. But she stopped short of pursuing her show business dreams because she was so embarrassed by her weight. Happily, through *The Biggest Loser*, Isabeau shed 113 pounds—and her fear of performing—and along with Hollie and Julie was one of three female finalists. Lighter and more confident, she's meeting with record executives and starting to sing professionally.

Julie Hadden: Runner-Up, Season 4

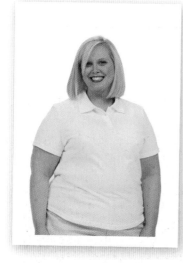

Before: 218 pounds
After: 121 pounds

Julie had always struggled with her weight. While growing up, she was known as the "chubby kid." As she got older, she began to lose weight and enter beauty pageants. But after the birth of her son, she had trouble shedding the baby weight and regaining her beauty queen body.

"Obviously, I knew I needed to lose weight or I wouldn't have auditioned for the show to begin with. But I have always hidden behind a big smile and covered everything up with black clothing to minimize my size. But still, I wasn't kidding myself about my problem."

When Julie started the show, she didn't even know how much she weighed. "They had kept our weight from us prior to the official weigh-in that was filmed for TV," she explains. "And to be honest—I know this sounds crazy—but I didn't know how big I was. We didn't have a scale in our home. And that was no accident."

When Julie saw her weight for the first time, she gasped at the number. Then she burst into tears. She had no idea it had gotten that out of control. "At that moment, I knew that I was there for a reason."

With a total weight loss of 97 pounds, Julie was Season 4's runner-up. Now she's living a healthy lifestyle again and is a fit, healthy role model for her son and her husband of 18 years.

Kae Whang

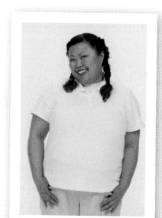

Before: 225 pounds
After: 128 pounds

Kae knows a thing or two about discipline—she is a former private in the US Army! She says that point in her life was the last time she was fit. But afterward, she started eating more fast food and stopped making the right choices. After years and years of an unhealthy diet, and without proper exercise, she kept growing. "You don't realize how quickly it happens," she says. "You're just in this denial stage, like, 'Oh, I'm not that big.' And then you go into this mentality that's like, 'Oh, I'll start tomorrow.' Well, tomorrow never really comes."

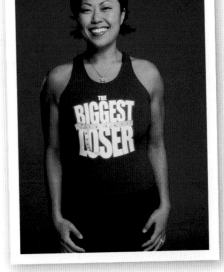

"When we first got to the ranch, and exercised with Bob, he told us, 'Remember how it feels to be this weight, and then later on keep reminding yourself how hard it is to be at this weight.' And boy, I will *never* forget how hard 225 pounds feels for a 5-foot, 2-inch person!"

Kae worked hard on *The Biggest Loser* to get back to her old self. She knew that if she lost weight and jumped on the road to a healthy lifestyle, she would regain the confidence she once had. And she did. She also did something no other woman on the show had ever done: She lost 20 pounds in 1 week. Now that's a testament to her commitment.

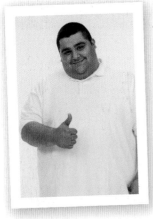

Neil Tejwani

Before: 421 pounds
After: 210 pounds

There was a time in Neil's life when he was athletic and participated in sports. But when he was 14, he broke his leg and couldn't play sports for a while, and he soon began gaining weight. Although Neil has a great job as a chemical engineer and an amazing girlfriend he hopes to spend many more years with, his health had been an obstacle. In fact, he was concerned about not reaching the age of 30.

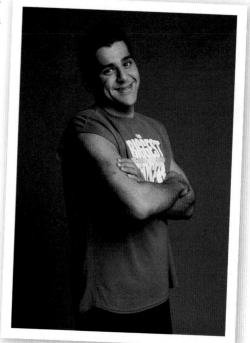

These days, Neil is the picture of health. "If you told me when I first started *The Biggest Loser,* that I would have lost 50 or 60 pounds, I would have been happy because, you know, that's 50 or 60 pounds in the right direction of where I need to be. But to lose over 100 pounds, lose 140 pounds? It's absolutely incredible. It's life changing."

After Neil was eliminated, he headed home and saw his family for the first time in months. "It was really an unbelievable experience," he recalls. "I had only seen my father cry once in his life, and he was definitely sobbing when he saw me. My parents had been so worried about my health for the longest time."

Now that he's lost so much weight, he has a renewed outlook on what looks to be a long and fulfilling life ahead of him. "With the progress I've made, I have no intention of letting myself slip because I've worked too hard to get this far."

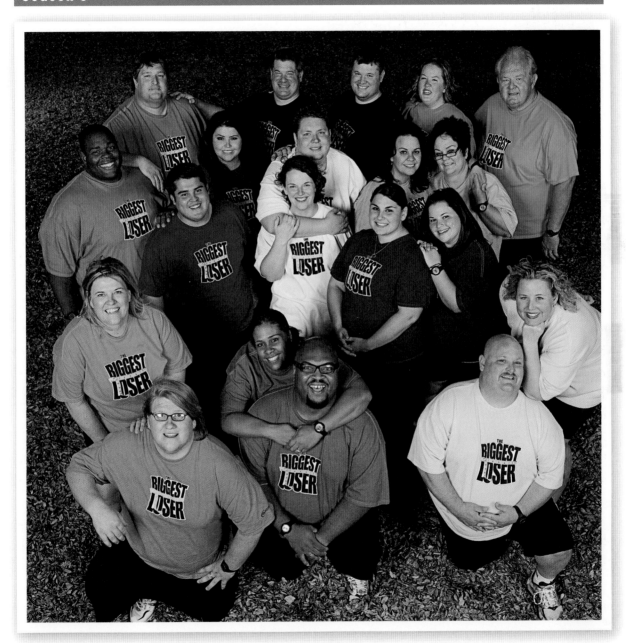

Ali Vincent

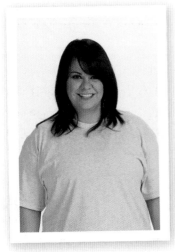

Starting weight: 234 pounds

This former champion synchronized swimmer was thin and fit until she quit her sport and stopped working out altogether. "I never really learned how to exercise," Ali confesses. "When I gained that first 5 pounds, I thought I was so fat!" Back then, stretch pants and sweaters were in, so Ali wore them to hide her body. But they hid her soaring weight even from her! By the time she reached her early 30s, she weighed well over 200 pounds—and climbing. This hairdresser from Arizona is working on getting down to a healthy weight, maintaining it, and not letting herself travel down Obesity Road. "I don't ever plan on being fat again," she vows.

One of Ali's hardest habits to overcome is frequenting restaurants and fast food places. "I'd have like four lattes a day, then a big meal at 10 o'clock at night. Every meal I had, I ate at a restaurant. It's a huge lifestyle change—but a change for the better."

Ali learned one very valuable new skill on *The Biggest Loser*: cooking. "When I got to the ranch, I didn't feel like I could prepare meals. But you have to cook if you want to eat there! I'm surprised at how well I cook now."

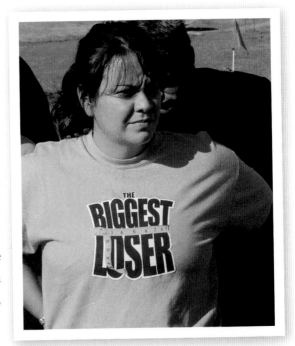

Ali is an outgoing, beautiful girl who is trapped inside her body. Her dream is to be an artist for a large corporation, but she knows she can't achieve her dream unless she loses the weight. Ali and her mom, Bette-Sue, partnered for Season 5.

Bette-Sue Burklund

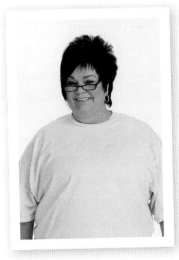

Starting weight: 261 pounds

As a motivational speaker for 20 years, Bette-Sue inspired people to change their lives, but deep down, she felt like a hypocrite because she couldn't get her weight under control. Having been a champion speed swimmer, she knows what she is capable of and what her body could look like if she could make a change. Bette-Sue is competitive to a fault and doesn't play unless she knows she can win.

Bette-Sue calls herself a "professional dieter." "I've been on every diet known to man and woman." But she vowed that *The Biggest Loser* plan would be the last one for her. Fortunately, she loves the meal plan. "I do like food, and that's the best part: I can eat and still lose weight."

At age 53, Bette-Sue takes pride in the fact that even though she was one of the oldest people on the ranch in Season 5, she lost weight faster than some of the younger women. In fact, she lost 37 pounds during her 4 weeks on the ranch! She thinks *The Biggest Loser* training is grueling. "I would fire a trainer who did that to me!" she declares. Bette-Sue wants her daughter and Season 5 partner, Ali, to lose weight so she will be happier. The two women are often mistaken for sisters, behave like siblings, and laugh out loud like children. Their relationship is special, though it's not without its difficulties.

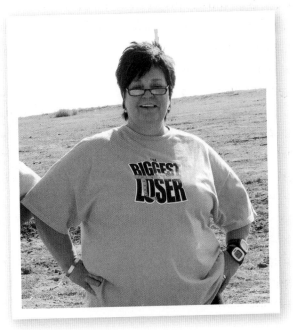

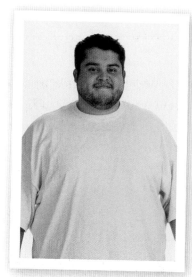

Bernie Salazar

Starting weight: 283 pounds

Selected from *The Biggest Loser* Online Club, this teacher led a sheltered life because he was too embarrassed by his weight to let himself be seen in public often. Overweight since the third grade, Bernie is the only chubby one in his family, and he's tired of it. He was never much of an exerciser, but now he's taken to it. Spinning is one of his favorites, and he sees himself biking along the lakefront in his hometown of Chicago. "Between finding exercise that I like and learning how to eat," he says, "I feel confident that I can reach my goal and stay there."

Bernie has a winning personality, and in the past he used his weight as a selling point. His name, *Bernardo*, Germanic in origin, is said to mean "brave as a bear." However, Bernie feels that a more appropriate translation of the name would be "heavy as a bear."

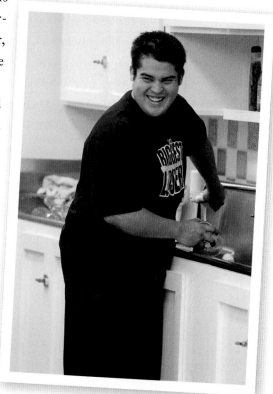

Five days a week, Bernie teaches English as a second language to parents in Chicago's Little Village community. "I have never said no to an opportunity and am continuously seeking ways to improve not only my life, but also the lives of my loved ones and those in my community," says Bernie. Even though he is healthy, Bernie is worried about his future. "My greatest fear is that my obesity will be the cause of an early death and I will be unable to attain my goals." For Season 5, Bernie teamed up with Brittany, a total stranger who quickly became a trusted ally.

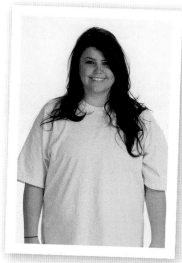

Brittany Aberle

Starting weight: 221 pounds

Brittany has been told she "has such a pretty face" for her whole life, and she's tired of it. She wants to hear "Damn, girl, you're hot!" Following in the footsteps of several women in her family, she decided to become a hairstylist. She thrives on being creative and making her clients feel beautiful. She is very strong willed, unafraid to say what's on her mind, and a true leader with a huge heart. A member of *The Biggest Loser* Online Club, Brittany was desperate to get a spot on the ranch and auditioned twice for previous seasons with no luck. They say the third time's a charm, and it was for Brittany. She was selected for the show as a single and paired up with another Club member, Bernie.

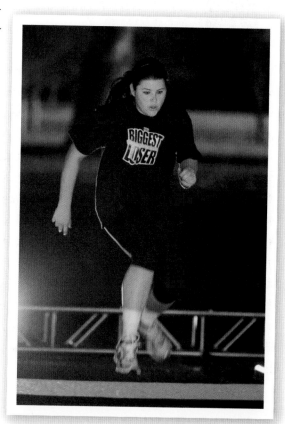

"I believe in not giving up!" she says. "It's such a blessing." She realizes that many people would like to be in her shoes. The exercises and physical challenges were a shock to her system, but she takes it all in stride, literally. "My muscles ache, but it's a good sore. I know my body is being put to the test," she says. By her 9th week at the ranch, Brittany had already lost 42 pounds!

Besides wanting to look good, Brittany has other reasons for getting in shape. "At age 22, I already have high blood pressure and high cholesterol. It's scary." Brittany derived a lot of encouragement and inspiration from the Biggest Loser trainers. "Their support really helps mentally, and their belief in my abilities is motivating."

She looks at food differently now, too. "A cheeseburger is 2 hours on the treadmill."

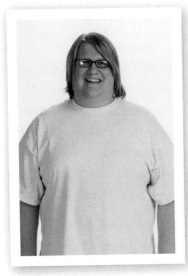

Dan Evans

Starting weight: 310 pounds

Dan is just a cool guy. He's really funny and very talented. He is an awesome rock and roll/country singer and believes his weight gets in the way of him achieving major success. Even though he hasn't yet found fame in Hollywood, he's attracting a growing number of fans.

For his full-time job, Dan works as a camp counselor for his family's business, a nonprofit after-school organization called Reach Out for Life Youth Foundation. There, he sings and entertains the kids whenever they give him a chance.

This singer-songwriter never saw the connection between eating and exercise until he got to the ranch; now he knows that you can burn off what you eat by working out, and that your diet also fuels you for exercise. "Understanding this principle was the key to my losing 91 pounds in the first 9 weeks," he says. "I have so much energy. I can't believe it." In the past, Dan shied away from the very thing he loves—performing onstage—due to his size. But now he has hope. "Even though I knew I was more than capable, I just wasn't confident about being in the spotlight. But now I feel more ready than I've ever felt before." Dan signed up for Season 5 with his mom, Jackie.

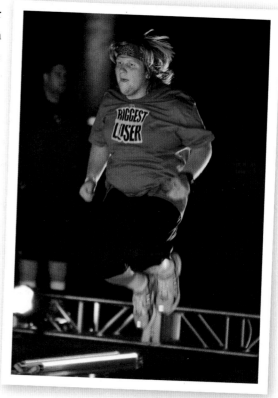

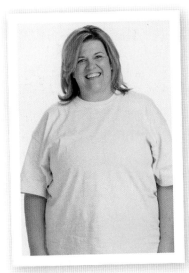

Jackie Evans

Starting weight: 246 pounds

Jackie has battled with her weight for her entire life. After getting married and having kids, she just kept gaining and gaining. No diet she tried ever worked. Discouraged, she developed a mind-set that was focused on failure and resigned herself to being fat. "I also knew I was getting older and that my metabolism was slowing down, making weight loss even more improbable," she says.

Jackie and her husband manage a nonprofit after-school organization that helps latchkey kids and at-risk youth stay safe. The program has been so successful that it's grown into a summer camp as well. But juggling the needs of 50 employees year-round leaves Jackie little time to cook healthful meals for her family, so they often eat out at their favorite restaurants. She realizes that she has raised her kids on unhealthy food, and she wants to start setting a better example.

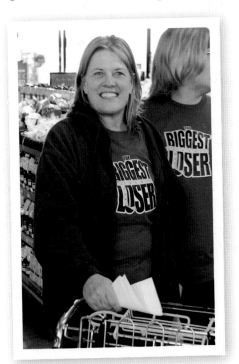

Jackie signed up for the show with the goal of getting healthy with her son. They were both shocked by how much their weight had soared when they first stepped onto the Biggest Loser scale and it registered a total of 556 pounds. Imagine her surprise when she started on *The Biggest Loser* and dropped 30 pounds in the first 3 weeks!

"What an eye-opener," she says. "There is no age barrier. It's about what you put in and what you put out." Eventually, she says, her goal is to fit into a little black dress and "feel sexy again."

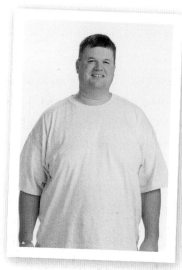

Jay Kruger

Starting weight: 293 pounds

"I always say I'm big boned, but I've never seen a fat skeleton," says Jay. He's been big all his life, but now it's becoming a problem. Concerned for Jay's health, his doctor recently advised him to either start losing weight or consider having gastric bypass surgery.

Jay is not a fan of exercise—he says his idea of fitness is riding in a golf cart for 18 holes—but he didn't want to have weight-loss surgery. Jay's motivation to do well on the show is to set a great example for his children and family. "The sun rises and sets on my kids, and I would go to the ends of the earth for them," he says.

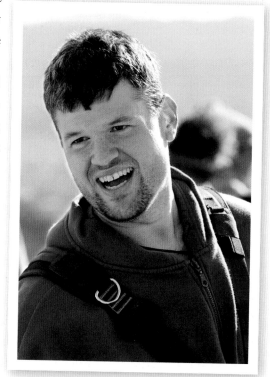

Jay has learned to trade in his doughnut-and-fast-food habits for a healthy diet of lean proteins, fruits, and vegetables ("But please, no quinoa!" he protests). He's eating between 1,800 and 2,000 calories a day—an amount that keeps him feeling full and satisfied. What most viewers don't realize is that contestants must cook their own food on the ranch; there's no personal chef, with the exception of Jay's personal chef, who is his brother and fellow team member, Mark. "Whatever he's cooking, I'm eating," Jay says.

Mark and Jay have a special bond and are often mistaken for twins. Through they come from a tight-knit family and do everything together, they are also competitive with one another and like to bust each other's chops.

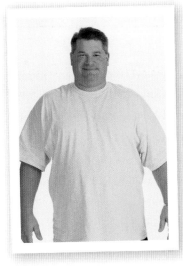

Mark Kruger

Starting weight: 285 pounds

Mark is a very approachable guy. He's honest and kind, and his sincere love for his family shows through whenever he speaks of them. Mark grew up as the middle child of three brothers. He believed he had to show off to stand out. He was very active in school and only gained the weight after he had a family.

Mark knew that his love of ice cream and his wife's great cooking were going to catch up with him sooner or later, so he's thankful to be a member of the Season 5 cast along with his brother, Jay. Though he is a very hard worker, Mark says he hasn't had time to really work out. He feels that the extra weight he carries is definitely keeping him from succeeding in his career, especially since his company encourages employees to be fit and healthy.

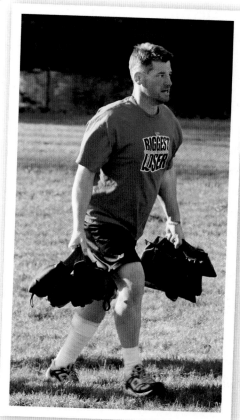

Since arriving at the ranch, though, Mark has noticed an internal change beginning to take place, in addition to the amazing physical changes that are more noticeable. "Our trainers do a great job of sitting us down and discussing emotional or mental issues that may have contributed to weight gain," he explains. "I'm strong emotionally, but I do have moments of weakness, like everybody does. I've always masked those by running to the refrigerator." Mark knows that getting a handle on emotional eating will ultimately translate into big losses on the scale.

Jenn Widder

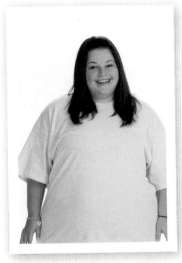

Starting weight: 254 pounds

Years ago, Jenn and her mother were driving up to the open house family weekend for Camp Shane (a weight-loss camp) and her mother said, "I hope we find it; I don't want to be late." Jenn remembers thinking to herself, "I hope we never find it."

Little did she know, however, that Camp Shane would be her home away from home for the next 10 summers and now her career of choice. She feels Camp Shane has definitely shaped her into the person she is today: incredibly outgoing, funny, and compassionate.

She says she auditioned for *The Biggest Loser* because "I am the assistant director for the most esteemed weight-loss camp in the country.

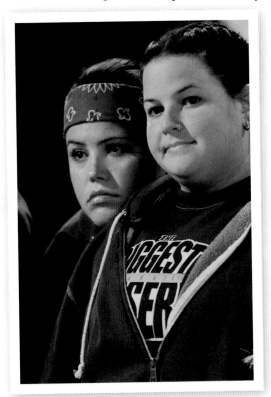

I have to lose weight. I am embarrassed. I am doing everything in my power to dodge questions like, 'Where are you working?' 'What are you doing with your life?' I want to be proud of me; I want for the first time to be able to be seen for who I am on the inside and outside. I want people to want to have a conversation with me because they find me to be interesting. I want this for me, and for no one else."

Dreams do come true. A fan of the show since Season 1, Jenn dreamed of being on *The Biggest Loser.* After being selected, Jenn knew that her life would be forever changed.

Jenn has a powerful can-do attitude, even in the face of her sluggish weight loss during the initial weeks of the show. "My numbers on the scale weren't the best, but I know I'm changing and I can see it in my face and when I look in the mirror . . . so I'm just gonna continue to stay positive," she says. Jenn paired up for the show with her best friend, Maggie.

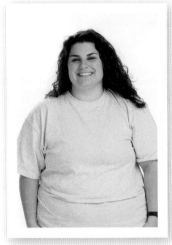

Maggie King

Starting weight: 239 pounds

Maggie is an outgoing, vivacious 23-year-old. When it comes to food, she says she's an emotional eater. "I eat when I'm feeling *any* emotion," she says. It doesn't help that she works as a restaurant server for part of the year, where she gets her food for free. "Thank God for Camp Shane, a weight-loss camp, where I have been both a camper and a staff member every summer for 11 years. I'd probably weigh 700 pounds by now if not for my time there!"

Maggie enjoys being around people and hanging out with friends. Since Maggie's been overweight all her life, she's learned to use humor as a distraction from her obesity. "People would describe me as 'the funny girl.' I've always been the 'best friend,' never the 'girlfriend'; I've never had a serious boyfriend although I would *love* one!"

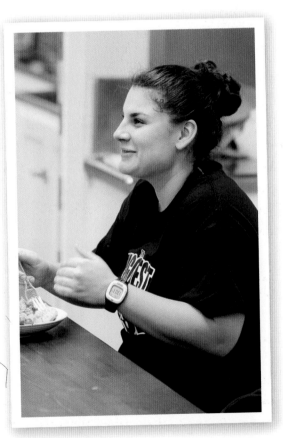

When her best pal, Jenn, invited her to audition for *The Biggest Loser*, Maggie was all for it. Then, when both girls made the cut, they were over-the-top excited. "Before being on the show, I thought I'd better get used to this because I'll never lose weight," she says. "After starting the program, I realized that I don't have to be fat forever."

Positive changes began happening right away. "Physically, I felt the best I had in a long time. I could breathe better. I could move better," Maggie says. "I feel successful every single day, and that's the best part. I am looking forward to living life as a thin person."

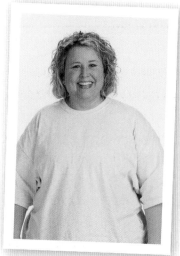

Kelly Fields

Starting weight: 271 pounds

Kelly wants nothing more than to have children, and she knows her weight could prevent her from realizing that dream. So Kelly decided to create her own destiny and lose the weight that is keeping her from the life she wants. She wanted to try out for Season 4 of *The Biggest Loser* but missed the application deadline. Disappointed but still determined, she decided to wait for the next season. So when NBC began casting for Season 5, Kelly had her audition tape ready and took it to the casting call in Miami.

Once she got there, she learned that the show was looking for pairs, so she called her ex-husband, Paul, to apply with her. Paul and Kelly met online 9 years ago and married shortly afterward. They were married for 7 years before divorcing and remained close friends. "This was the opportunity of a lifetime," Kelly says. "I'd made up my mind that if I didn't get on the show, I had to do something somehow. My doctor was ready to prescribe weight-loss medication for me."

Learning about portion control, calorie counting, and high-intensity exercise has started to reshape Kelly's body and life. She began her stint on the ranch as the "biggest girl in the house" but was soon on her way to becoming one of the sexiest.

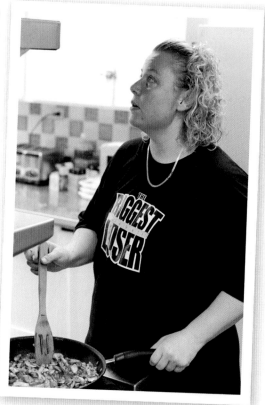

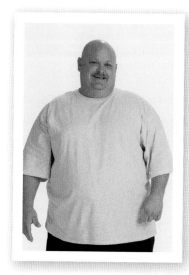

Paul Marks

Starting weight: 303 pounds

Paul is a big teddy bear of a man. He'd love nothing more than to get fit and healthy. An ex-soldier with a heart of gold, Paul always roots for the underdog—probably because he is one of them.

As a bachelor over the past few years, Paul hasn't done much cooking. He tended to eat convenient grab-and-go foods like pizza and fried chicken, and he'd reheat the leftovers from his junk-food dinners for breakfast and lunch, as well—a habit that sent his weight soaring to 303 pounds. Because contestants must prepare their own meals at the ranch, Paul has begun to learn new cooking techniques and healthy versions of his favorite recipes, and he is starting to actually enjoy being in the kitchen. "Cooking food here is easier than I expected—and it tastes great!" he says.

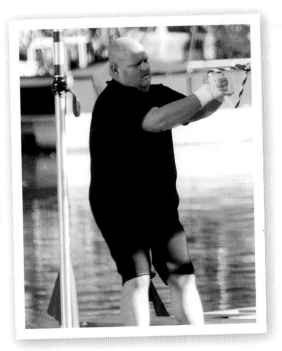

Sure, Paul knows there's a cash prize of $250,000 dangling out there like a huge carrot, but he knows he's already a winner. "I feel energetic and youthful again, and I'm doing things athletically I haven't done in years," he says.

At 43, Paul's main concern with being overweight is his family history of bad health. His dad died at age 47, his grandfather at age 49, and his great grandfather at age 51. Paul is determined to break that trend.

Roger Shultz

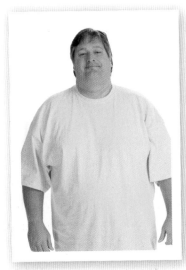

Starting weight: 363 pounds

When Roger walks into a room, you can see his personality from a mile away. A live sports radio host, he's very proud of his own college career in football at the University of Alabama. Seeing his college pictures will tell you why—the guy was hot! He's very passionate about getting back to his playing weight, not only for his health, but also because he wants to look like his twin brother again, who weighs 198 pounds. Roger is paired with one of his old football buddies, Trent, for Season 5.

Roger auditioned for *The Biggest Loser* Season 3 but wasn't selected for the show. Not willing to give up, he auditioned for Season 4, but didn't make the cut that time, either. Much to his surprise, he got a call to see if he'd be interesting in being on Season 5. He told the casting director: "Well, I'm still fat, so yes, I'm available."

When Roger and his wife got married, he weighed 383 pounds—and he has hated his wedding pictures ever since because he was so fat. "I've set a goal to take my wife dancing," he says. "In fact, that's the goal I inscribed on my flag at the ranch. I'm planning on putting on a tux, taking her dancing, and having a really great picture of us taken—with me thin!"

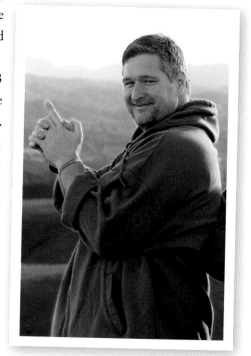

After his first 10 days on the ranch, something amazing happened to Roger, a type 2 diabetic who was taking an oral diabetes drug: He was told he could discontinue taking his medicine. "My blood sugar is better than it's ever been, better than when I was taking medicine. It's unbelievable," he says. Naturally, that made a believer out of this former football player, who went on to lose almost 100 pounds during his first 9 weeks at the ranch.

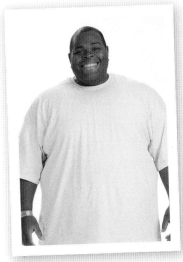

Trent Patterson

Starting weight: 436 pounds

Trent is a lovable guy with a great smile. But you can tell that beneath that soft exterior lies a fierce competitor. He's very passionate about his wife, their new family . . . and food.

As a University of Alabama football player, Trent ate yards of food but easily burned it off with his intense training regimen. He stopped playing football but didn't stop eating all that food, and the fat piled on—all 436 pounds of it. "My buddy Roger called me and asked me how much I weighed. I told him I was 436 and he said, 'Good.' I wondered what could be so good about that, and Roger told me *The Biggest Loser* was looking for really heavy pairs to be on in Season 5. We auditioned, and the rest is history," Trent recalls.

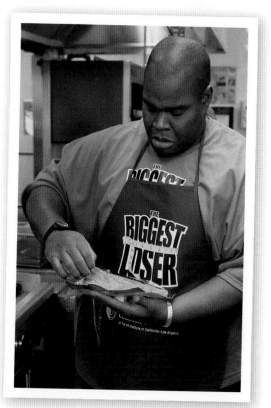

Friends for 20 years, Trent backs up his partner Roger 100 percent. They talk about their football training camp like they've been through war.

These likeable cast members are used to having their butts whipped into shape from their harsh training back in their glory days. In fact, Trent says their college football camp days make Biggest Loser workouts look easy!

Once he started on a low-calorie diet, began training almost as hard as in his football days, and limiting his intake to about 2,200 calories per day, Trent shed 87 pounds during his 7 weeks on the ranch—and is motivated to keep losing. "This is a new beginning for me," he says.

In addition to your favorite Biggest Losers, you'll meet eight inspiring people from *The Biggest Loser* Online Club (www.biggestloserclub.com) who have transformed themselves at home by using the very same strategies that cast members employ. They are people just like you, and they'll be sharing their real-world tips and encouragement along with the cast members. They're living proof that, with healthful nutrition, doable workouts, and the will to succeed, you can reach your weight-loss goal and stay there!

There you have it—ordinary people who have managed to lose huge amounts of weight and are living a completely transformed lifestyle as a result. As you read their stories and strategies, you'll find that a positive mental outlook and dedication are just as important as calorie counting and cardio. Poor health habits and the problems they bring can only begin to change when you change your attitude, and these Biggest Losers will help you do that. You'll find, as they did, that your feelings of self-worth will improve as the pounds fall off.

The Biggest Losers will share their amazing strategies for:

- Galvanizing your desire to get healthy with the power of a transformative moment

- Handling cravings, emotional eating, and over-indulgence with psychological techniques

- Developing the staying power needed to start and maintain an exercise program you can live with and love—even if you think you hate to exercise, like many of the contestants did

- Loving yourself to good health, so you can build a better body, a more attractive appearance, self-confidence, and renewed energy

- Building a support network that will keep you focused, motivated, and healthy for a lifetime

- Living fit and staying fit so you'll never have to wrestle with obesity again

The journey to a more slender, healthy body isn't always easy. But luckily for you, the Biggest Losers are sharing their road map. As you begin to employ their strategies and feel inspired by their stories, the old, unhealthy you will start to fade, and you'll have a fresh, new start on life. Although only a handful of people can win the coveted title of "The Biggest Loser," everyone can shed unwanted pounds and win this valuable prize—a healthier, more fulfilling life!

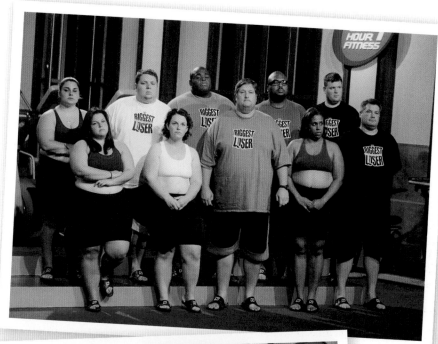

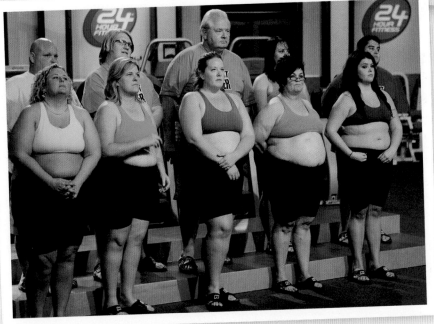

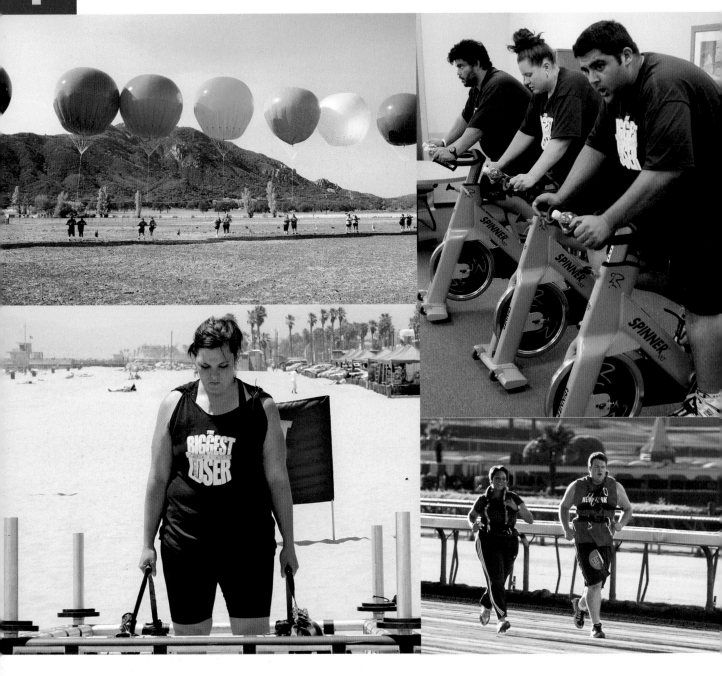

1

The Inspiration to Make a Change: Getting Started

Y ou may be surprised to learn that one of the most important components of a weight-loss strategy isn't grit-your-teeth willpower or having the latest, greatest exercise machine. It's not even coming into this world with the right genes. It's being motivated to make lasting changes in your life. A lot of people refer to this as their "moment," and every single Biggest Loser on NBC's mega-hit show has had one. For each of them, it was the kicking-off point for losing weight and staying dedicated to their goals.

This moment—which researchers call a "triggering event"—could be the result of a frightening medical diagnosis, an emotional struggle, or a sudden, life-changing event. Whatever form it takes, your moment is something that causes you to reevaluate your life and your choices from a new perspective and motivates you to

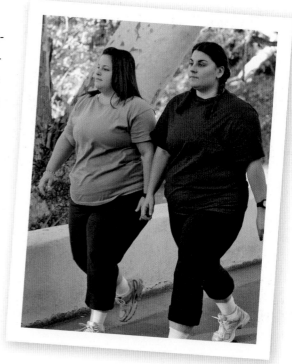

take charge of your own destiny. So the next time someone makes a rude comment about your weight or your doctor warns you that your health is in danger, be grateful. Their words may be just what you need to get started.

In this chapter you will read about the moments that moved some of your favorite Biggest Losers to action. They all experienced a turning point that made them realize their lifestyle was no longer acceptable and that changes—big changes—were in order. Their stories may be just what *you* need to get inspired and change your life forever.

Neil Tejwani, Season 4: "The desire to make a long, happy life with the woman I love was my moment."

Sometimes the motivation to change your life doesn't come from you, but from the concern and coaxing of a loved one. Such was the case with Neil, who eventually found his weight-loss inspiration in his relationship with his girlfriend, Steph. She wanted him to lose weight and nudged him gently to do so because she feared for his health. That was his first big moment. Then he learned that his life was truly in jeopardy because of his weight. That was his second moment. Here is his story.

"I tipped the scales at 460 pounds—the heaviest I've ever been," he explains. "My doctor told me that I would not live to see the age of 30—a strain that came between Steph and me. She had been very scared that I might die, so we never made plans to get married, although we had been together for 5 years and were very much in love."

Neil decided to look into gastric bypass surgery. He trudged through all the required classes, psychological evaluations, and group meetings. "It was a long, tedious process, and to be honest, my heart was really never in it," Neil says. "But my father, who is a doctor, sat me down and said, 'Look, you're 25 years old and the path you're going down is a recipe for disaster. I'm not sure you even have a future.'"

Hearing those harsh words from his father cinched Neil's decision to have the surgery. In preparation, he was instructed to lose 10 percent of his body weight—a little more than 40 pounds.

He started exercising 30 minutes a day on a recumbent bike and eating healthier. He took the 40 pounds off. "The success I had gave me the confidence to continue losing weight on my own. I felt I could do it without surgery. A psychologist at the hospital told me I'd eventually gain it back—and that I needed the surgery to keep off the weight long-term. I'm very competitive, and when someone tells me I can't do something, I make it happen. I told the psychologist that the next time he saw me, I would have lost weight on my own, and I walked out of his office."

At about that time, Steph, who has always been a fan of *The Biggest Loser*, encouraged Neil to answer a casting call for Season 4. He never dreamed he'd have a chance, but he went for it anyway. "I wanted an opportunity to change my life," he says. "*The Biggest Loser* gave me that opportunity. I've taken off more than 200 pounds since starting the program. The look of worry is finally gone from her face, and that's a great feeling for me."

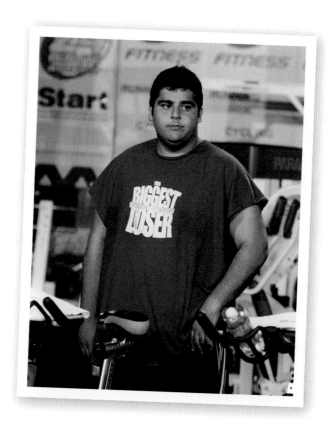

Kelly Fields, Season 5: "I didn't want to be insignificant anymore."

Kelly's story speaks to the heart of every woman who has ever struggled with her weight. At 271 pounds, she says, "I was really tired of being overweight. There were so many limitations. I couldn't cross my legs. I'd have to assess a chair before I sat down. I couldn't go through a turnstile—not even sideways. I had to use the handicapped stalls in bathrooms; normal stalls were too small for me. Most people just don't know how hard and inconvenient it is to be so heavy."

Kelly hid her body beneath nice clothes she bought at a department store that carried her size, and she says it worked. "A lot of people told me, 'You don't need to lose weight.' But the reality of her weight problem began creeping up on her. One day she discovered that even the department store's largest size wasn't fitting anymore. She knew her problem was getting worse.

But the real turning point came while Kelly was at work. The head nurse at a heart catheter-

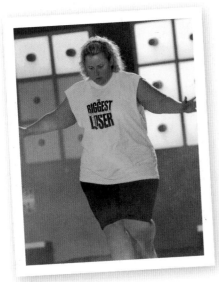

ization lab, Kelly had always taken pride in the fact that she was the go-to person who could solve any problem—it was something she excelled at. But when a new nurse joined her team, Kelly says she began to feel less important. "She was gorgeous, with a beautiful figure and long blonde hair. I bet she didn't weigh an ounce over 130 pounds. She was so stunning that people would trip over themselves to say hi to her while ignoring me. I began to notice how insignificant I was. I didn't exist.

"That's when it really hit me hard: I've got to do something about my weight. I was done with being fat." Kelly's desire to feel confident and be noticed motivated her to try out for *The Biggest Loser*. She was tired of feeling insignificant.

"It was the opportunity of a lifetime when I was selected," she says. "When I started, I was the biggest girl in the house. Now I'm exercising and eating healthy foods. I've learned that my weight was a shell in which I could hide. I'm on a journey back to significance."

Dan Evans, Season 5: "A close friend of mine died at age 21."

For Dan, the death of a close friend triggered his moment. All of his friend's medical problems could have been prevented by living a healthier lifestyle. Dan realized that if he didn't improve his own health, he might suffer the same fate. Any health-related crisis is a powerful impetus for change. In fact, a study published in Preventive Medicine *found that people who were motivated by such an event were able to successfully lose weight.*

Dan had tried out for Season 4 of *The Biggest Loser* and was chosen as an alternate. When he wasn't picked to be on the show, he was very disappointed. "I went into a real funk because I had put so much into it," he recalls. "I was just coming out of that funk when I got the shocker of my life: My friend had died of a heart attack. He was only 21, like me. And he was overweight . . . like me. The doctors said his arteries were clogged."

In a positive twist of fate, *The Biggest Loser* called Dan shortly after his friend's death to ask if he'd be interested in trying out for Season 5. He says, "The timing was perfect. My friend's death scared me, and I sure didn't want to head down that road."

For Dan, being on *The Biggest Loser* represented a once-in-a-lifetime chance not only to change his health, but also to make his show business dreams come true. "Music is my thing," he says. "I love singing and playing the guitar, and I've done live stage musicals. But I've always been inhibited about performing, even though I know I've got talent. Who would want to look at some 310-pound guy onstage?"

Dan simply wasn't comfortable in his own skin. But now that's changing. He lost 91 pounds in the first 9 weeks at the ranch. And while his weight is on the way down, his confidence is on the way up. "When I return home, I'm going to take my career more seriously. I know what I want to do with my life—and I want to do it thin."

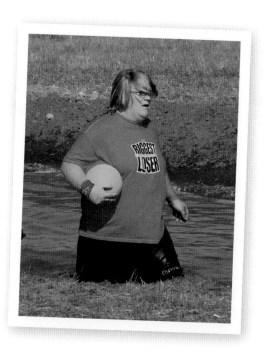

Bernie Salazar, Season 5: "I want to get back in the game of life."

Bernie's story illustrates how positive role models can help you make positive changes. Surrounding yourself with people who are committed to having a healthy lifestyle is a powerful motivator. They make fitness look achievable and appealing, and you want to join in. That's how Bernie, age 27, turned his life around.

Overweight all his life, Bernie was unable to do half of the things his friends were doing. He was too self-conscious to go to the beach and take his shirt off in public. He avoided restaurants because he didn't want people to see him eating. He was petrified to even walk into a gym, so he never exercised. Bernie became a near-recluse, rarely venturing anywhere for fear of being stared at.

But deep down, he had always wanted to keep

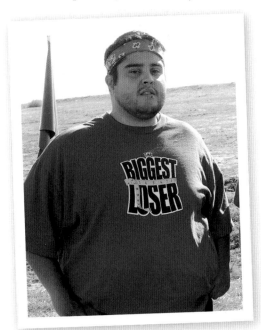

up with his family, all of whom are physically fit and active. "My younger brother is going to Disney World to run a marathon, and my family is going with him," Bernie says. "That's the kind of trip my family often takes—and I'm usually the guy holding the map instead of joining in. I'm tired of it."

Wanting to join in the fun with his healthy family finally made Bernie say, "Enough is enough." He had placed too much of his life on hold because of his weight. After he was selected for the show from *The Biggest Loser* Online Club, Bernie's life began to change. He started the show at 283 pounds and lost 82 pounds in the first 9 weeks. At 5 feet 5 inches tall, he's aiming for a goal weight of 140 or 145.

"I feel like the rest of my life is pretty well put together," he says. "I have a very supportive family. I have a beautiful girlfriend who is 100 percent behind me, too. I just completed my master's in education. I've been able to successfully manage every aspect of my life—except my weight. But now that's changing."

Isabeau Miller, Season 4: "My life just wasn't working."

At 21 years old and almost 300 pounds, Isabeau knew she needed to do something about her weight, especially since she is a singer-songwriter in the very image-based entertainment industry.

Because of her size, Isabeau put her career on the back burner. You've heard the expression "It's not over until the fat lady sings"; well, this singer isn't fat anymore, and she's ready to begin her new life. Encouraged by her experience on *The Biggest Loser*, she's not ashamed to be onstage again. Her story is a testament to what can happen if you put your mind to losing weight and stay focused on changing your life.

"No one can prepare you for the emotion when someone basically gives you a second chance on your life, as *The Biggest Loser* did for me," she recalls. "When I was told I was going to be on the show, I was just overcome with emotion. I felt like someone offered to save my life. Yes, I was absolutely nervous about losing weight on national TV. But I looked at it as an opportunity to show America, my family, and myself what I was at my absolute worst so I could only get better from there. It was a matter of pride for me."

Isabeau has lost 113 pounds. Originally, she went into the process looking for inspiration from outside sources, such as her teammates, family, and friends. But she learned something more valuable: "Ultimately, the greatest lesson I learned is to

look inside yourself for inspiration. I want to be the best me I can be. That's what keeps me going. It used to be that I wanted to wear cute clothes, to go shopping anywhere, and other external reasons for weight loss. But in the end, it's that I want to live the longest, healthiest, best life I can. That's what keeps me going."

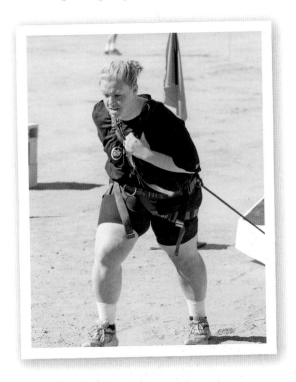

Kae Whang, Season 4: "I was tired of being ashamed of myself."

A powerful emotion—such as shame—often triggers an intense desire to change. That's what happened to Kae. Her story is a hopeful message about overcoming years of shame-filled living by channeling all of that negative energy in a more positive direction.

"I couldn't do the littlest things, like tie my shoe," Kae recalls. "With every move I made, breathing was a struggle. I was too embarrassed to even think about going to my high school reunion. I was too ashamed of how I looked to visit my family in Korea. A lot of things were conspiring against me. I asked myself if I was happy, and the answer was no. The shame I felt was my wake-up call."

Kae was petrified about losing weight on national television. "I didn't want people to see me in my bra and spandex, with the fat and stretch marks I had been hiding for most of my life."

But losing 20 pounds in the first week inspired Kae to keep going and going. Getting good results at first is common, and Kae was able to use this initial push to create healthy new habits that saw her through when that "high" wore off. She eventually lost 97 pounds at the ranch.

Now Kae is planning something she had put off for 20 years—a visit to her homeland of Korea. "I am determined to get on that plane," she says. "I feel like I can do anything now."

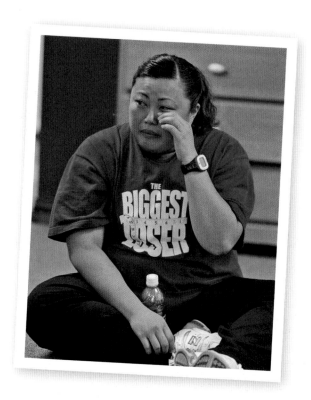

Amy Hildreth, Season 3: "I couldn't catch my breath walking up stairs."

Overweight when she was growing up, Amy was pressured by her parents to slim down. They wanted the best for her, and it was hard for them to see Amy getting bigger each year. They were concerned for her health as well as her social life, but the approach they took was one that eventually ended up hurting Amy more deeply than they ever intended. The many arguments over her weight made the teenage Amy rebellious. She wasn't going to let anyone tell her she wasn't okay the way she was, and to prove it, she just began to eat more. And more. And more.

As Amy got older, she became aware that something had to change. She was no longer happy with the way she was and knew that her weight was affecting her life more than she had ever thought it would. "When I started working in a sales job, I put on another 40 pounds. I got to the point where I couldn't walk up a flight of stairs without being out of breath," she explains. "That was my moment. I knew I really needed help. I was only 26 years old."

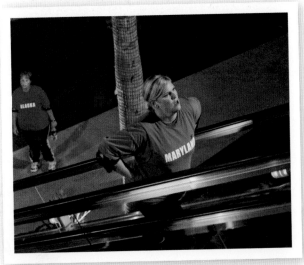

To break free of the chubby-girl identity and move in a healthier direction, she stood in line for hours among 1,200 people for a chance to change her life with *The Biggest Loser*. And it paid off.

Amy started on *The Biggest Loser* at 260 pounds, and she was so out of shape that she was afraid to exercise. Trainer Bob Harper's goal was to get her running.

"One day we were running to the gate and back," says Amy. "I felt so exhausted I couldn't move. Bob asked me, 'What are you afraid of?' And he was right, I *could* keep running, but I just needed someone to tell me it's okay to push myself. I conquered my fear of pushing myself during workouts."

By the finale, Amy weighed 180 pounds. And she has not only overcome her fear of physical activity, exercise is now her profession and her passion. She and her fiancé, fellow *Biggest Loser* contestant Marty Wolff, became certified as personal trainers by the American Council on Exercise and started a business called Reality Wellness so they could help others.

Jenn Widder, Season 5: "Someone told me I was fat, and it hurt."

Jenn is a counselor at a summer camp called Camp Shane, which is a weight-loss camp for children. One day, she brought in a celebrity for a personal appearance. The celebrity blurted out to Jenn, "You're beautiful. You have so much going for you, but you're really overweight."

"Her bluntness was a pivotal, rock-bottom moment in my life because nobody, except my parents, had ever said that to me," Jenn says. "And I knew that whether I got on the show or not, this year would be the year that I finally lost weight.

"I thought that working at a weight-loss camp would help me with my own weight, but it didn't turn out that way. Although I love that job, it's unsettling to me to be overweight and be the assistant director of a weight-loss camp. What an oxymoron! When camp starts up again in the summer, I'm going to have 550 kids who hopefully will be motivated and inspired by my story. I think about that every day. Every time I get on the scale, I tell myself I'm doing it for those kids—and for me." During her stay at *The Biggest Loser* ranch, Jenn lost 31 pounds, and she is looking forward to losing even more.

Hearing a negative comment about your weight sticks with you—but it can also help you stick with a program to lose weight, as it did for Jenn. She used it as motivation to make a plan not only for losing weight, but for keeping it off permanently.

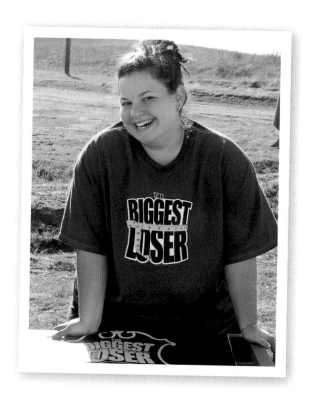

David Griffin, Season 4: "I don't want to cheat my wife and kids."

The desire to be there for your family—and do things with them—is another top motivator for successful weight loss. You want to live longer and be more active, not just for yourself, but for your spouse and your children. That's how David became so single-minded about losing weight. His family was energetic and full of life—and he couldn't keep up with them.

"My moment occurred when day-to-day activities like walking to my barn or playing with my kids became impossible to do without feeling tired and out of breath," he says. "My weight was holding me back from life."

David also knew that he was at risk for a variety of weight-related health problems, including hypertension and high cholesterol. He was aware that these conditions could sneak up on him and lead to life-threatening diseases, and he didn't want to leave his family. So David made a decision to be there for them in every way. When he auditioned for *The Biggest Loser*, he was only 32 and already weighed 368 pounds.

"I have constant reminders every day of why I have to be healthy: my wife and my children," David says. "I don't want to cheat them. Now I can work out for an hour and a half a day like normal people do, and I make sure my kids absolutely know how important it is to eat healthy and to exercise." And instead of struggling to keep up with the pack, David now leads the family with his own healthy example. "Our kids go to the gym with us and play basketball," he says. "We just signed our 3-year-old up for indoor soccer for the winter. I have a huge passion not only for my family, but for anyone who is out of shape. I hope I'm setting a great example, because I really want to see America become healthier."

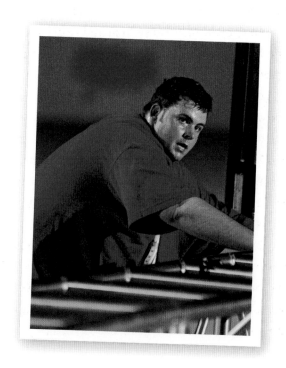

Paul Marks, Season 5: "I was taking five drugs for high blood pressure."

Paul didn't want to join the long list of men in his family who had died young. His doctor had already diagnosed him with malignant hypertension, which is extremely high blood pressure that can lead to stroke, kidney failure, or heart failure. If malignant hypertension isn't treated, the person's life expectancy can be as short as 2 years. Paul was put on five drugs to manage his dangerously high blood pressure. And he was alarmed to discover that at age 42, he couldn't even qualify for life insurance after getting that diagnosis. He knew he had to do something about his weight, but he wasn't sure where to start.

His ex-wife, Kelly, told him that *The Biggest Loser* was casting pairs for Season 5. She was in Miami auditioning and was asked if she knew anyone who'd be interested in doing the show with her. She said, "The only other fat person I know is my ex-husband." This piqued the interest of the casting director.

Kelly called Paul and said, "To get onto the ark, you have to go two by two. Are you interested?" He was.

"Fortunately or unfortunately, Kelly had a picture of me, wearing a Speedo, on her digital camera," Paul says. "As soon as the casting director saw the photo, he wanted to interview me—I guess I looked pretty bad. The *Biggest Loser* staff met with us for 2 hours, and they liked our odd dynamic of bickering back and forth. We were cast for the show, and the roller coaster started."

Paul began *The Biggest Loser* weighing 303 pounds, and he lost 67 pounds during his 8 week stay. With healthful eating and regular exercise, he was able to discontinue all five blood pressure medicines.

"It is a miracle," he says. "I feel energetic and youthful again. I'm literally saving my life."

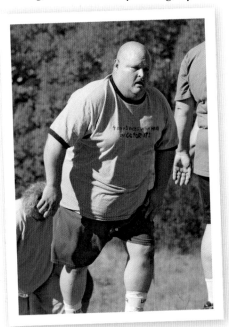

The Biggest Loser Online Club Profile: **Theresa Pucket**

Starting weight: 240 • Current weight: 165 • Goal weight: 145–150

Heavy most of her life, Theresa's first moment of realization came when her mother-in-law, who is diabetic, had one of her legs amputated.

"At that point, seeing what my mother-in-law went through, I realized that I really needed to do something about my weight or I would be facing the same fate.

"I had tried to 'diet' many times during my life, but I just never really had the motivation needed to stick with it."

So in September of 2003, weighing in at an all-time high of 250 pounds, Theresa started a low-carb diet. She did well for the first four months but eventually lost momentum and gained the weight back. "I stuck my head in the sand, put away the scale, and refused to face my failure," she recalls.

A couple of years later, her husband took a picture of her that shattered her world. "When I got the film developed, I nearly cried. Stepping back on the scale, I found myself 10 pounds shy of my highest weight."

Theresa began browsing the Internet for answers and received an e-mail advertising *The Biggest Loser* Online Club. She checked out the site and found what she didn't want to hear but knew she needed: a program that wasn't a "diet" at all, but a total lifestyle change incorporating healthy eating, calorie control, and exercise. No magic pills, no easy out, just hard work, personal accountability, and sweat! Theresa signed up and made a commitment to change her life.

"*The Biggest Loser* Online Club has helped me to become a totally new person," she says. "I am now so much more active than I ever was before. I used to spend most of my day sitting, usually reading."

Theresa devised motivational strategies to help her stay focused. "I took monthly pictures of myself and posted them on the wall above my scale. Seeing the physical changes in me from month to month has helped tremendously. I also posted a list of all the reasons why I wanted to lose weight; then after a time I started a new list of the ways my life has improved. When I hit rough patches, I go back to those pictures and lists.

"The best advice I can give is to take it one day at a time, one pound at a time, and make this a lifetime commitment to health!"

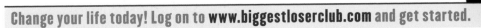

Change your life today! Log on to www.biggestloserclub.com and get started.

Are You Ready? 10 Steps to Get Started

Maybe you've experienced your own life-changing moment, or perhaps one of the stories in this chapter clicked with you. Just knowing that you're ready to get started is an important accomplishment. If you feel that fire in your belly, here are a few guidelines from *The Biggest Loser* for getting started now.

Step 1: Admit you have a weight problem.

If you're overweight, fess up! Denial can prevent you from taking action and pounds will keep piling on, leading to health problems and more weight that will have to come off down the road. Says Kelly Fields, Season 5: "When I saw pictures of myself, I realized how heavy I had gotten. I had to face the music."

Step 2: Don't make excuses.

There's never a "good" time to start a weight-loss program. Just ask the contestants, who leave their jobs and families for several months to be at the ranch. The time to start living healthfully is *now*—whether it's convenient or not.

Step 3: Learn from your past.

Most people have been on umpteen diets. Okay, maybe you failed in the past, but use this as an opportunity to learn from your mistakes. What worked for you before? What didn't work? What did you like about one diet or hate about another? Incorporate your strengths into your new diet plan and try to avoid things that tripped you up in the past.

Step 4: Make a clean sweep of all junk food.

You can't eat it if it's not there! Rid your environment—home, office, car—of foods that aren't nutritious or that will cause you to overeat. Replace problem foods with healthy choices such as those recommended on *The Biggest Loser* diet, including fresh fruits, vegetables, whole grains, fish, lean meats and poultry, and low-fat dairy products.

Step 5: Build your team.

"Everybody's got to have a really strong support group if they're going to get healthy," says David Griffin, Season 4. "There has to be at least one person who is willing to go that mile with you. For me, that's my wife."

Toughest Moment: Bernie Salazar, Season 5

Realizing just how much of my life I had placed on hold because of my weight.

The research shows clearly that people who lose weight and keep it off have good support systems to help them along. So start recruiting a team to help keep you on track. This could be your family, your coworkers, a personal trainer, an exercise partner, a running or hiking club, an online support group on www.biggestloserclub.com, or a weight-loss group. No matter what form it takes, having support will help you stay on track and strengthen your resolve.

Step 6: Set realistic goals.

You've heard it a million times, but if your goals aren't realistic and attainable, you'll get frustrated and most likely quit. Set small goals that you can meet each week to maintain your enthusiasm and momentum. If you need help setting appropriate goals for your age and body weight, talk to your doctor or a registered dietitian.

Step 7: Make daily resolutions toward reaching your goals.

Early in a program to change your lifestyle, it's helpful to make daily resolutions that are manageable rather than focusing on far-off end goals. Your daily resolutions should be a cinch to pull off. Focus on small steps, like eating two extra servings of vegetables, learning a new exercise, walking for an extra 30 minutes, and playing an active game with the kids. If all you do is concentrate on what you need to do today, achieving your end goal—like losing 50 pounds or fitting into size 6 jeans—will take care of itself. That's exactly what the Biggest Losers do every day at the ranch—concentrate on what they must do that day.

Step 8: Set your calorie budget.

On the show, each cast member's calorie limit is determined by a formula that considers his or her starting weight, body-fat percentage, and goal weight. Kae Whang, Season 4, for example, first weighed in at 230 pounds and follows a 1,200-calorie-a-day diet, while Isabeau Miller, Season 4, who started at almost 300 pounds, eats between 1,500 and 1,600 calories daily.

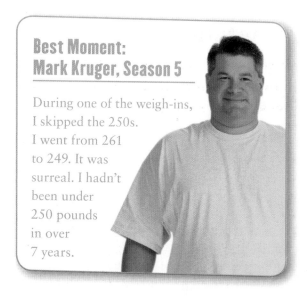

**Best Moment:
Mark Kruger, Season 5**

During one of the weigh-ins, I skipped the 250s. I went from 261 to 249. It was surreal. I hadn't been under 250 pounds in over 7 years.

At home, use this simple formula to determine your limits: If you are obese and sedentary, multiply your goal weight by 10 as a starting point. So, for instance, if you want to get down to 135 pounds, eat about 1,350 calories a day. If you're fairly active, multiply by 13 per pound, for about a 1,755-calorie allowance to reach 135. Keep in mind that additional variables may factor in, as well, such as gender and age, which may increase or decrease your budget slightly.

Step 9: Plan to be active for at least 60 minutes a day.

"Before I got here, I imagined we'd start with 20 minutes one day, maybe 40 minutes the next," laughs Isabeau. "Ha!" Biggest Losers jump right in, with cardio training lasting for hours at a time. Should you do the same? No. Contestants are pushed to work out harder than average, but only because they are under the close supervision of trainers and a medical staff. What *you* can do safely to reach your own fitness goal is to shoot for 60 minutes of physical activity a day at a moderately intense level. (If you're over age 50 or have a chronic disease or are at risk of developing one, consult your doctor before starting any plan.)

Step 10: Expect to have setbacks.

Cheryl Forberg, RD, nutritionist to *The Biggest Loser* cast, says that change doesn't come without setbacks. "If you slip up today, jump back in the game tomorrow by eating less, exercising more, or both. With a little motivation and dedication, you'll find yourself fit and full of energy this year. Losing weight may be just a bonus."

Adds Bernie Salazar, Season 5: "Love the small steps forward you're taking, and love the small steps backward you're taking because that's what makes you, you. Don't let those discourage you. Tomorrow is a new day."

As these stories show, the real challenge in transformation is not only figuring out what to do, it's having the courage and the drive to actually do it. If you're ready to get on the right road and get a fresh start in life, read on. By following the success strategies gleaned from five seasons of *The Biggest Loser*, you'll begin living a healthier, happier life—starting now.

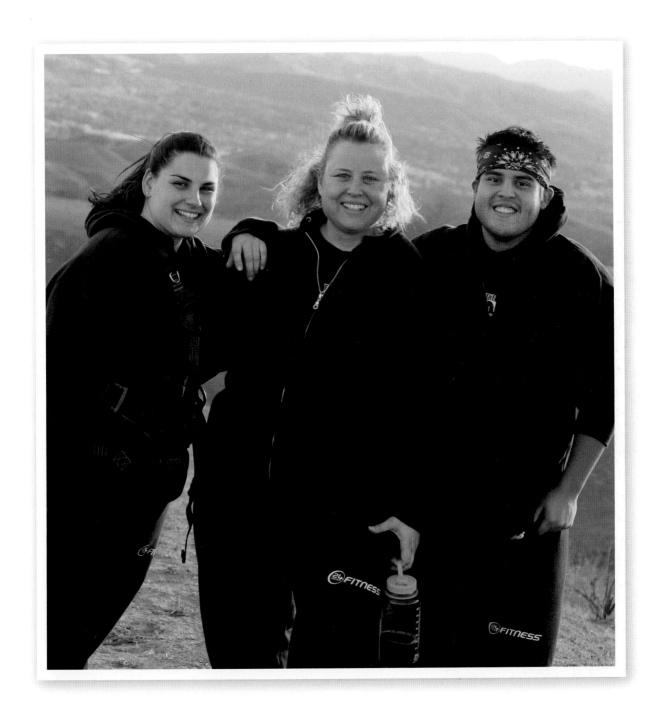

THE INSPIRATION TO MAKE A CHANGE: GETTING STARTED

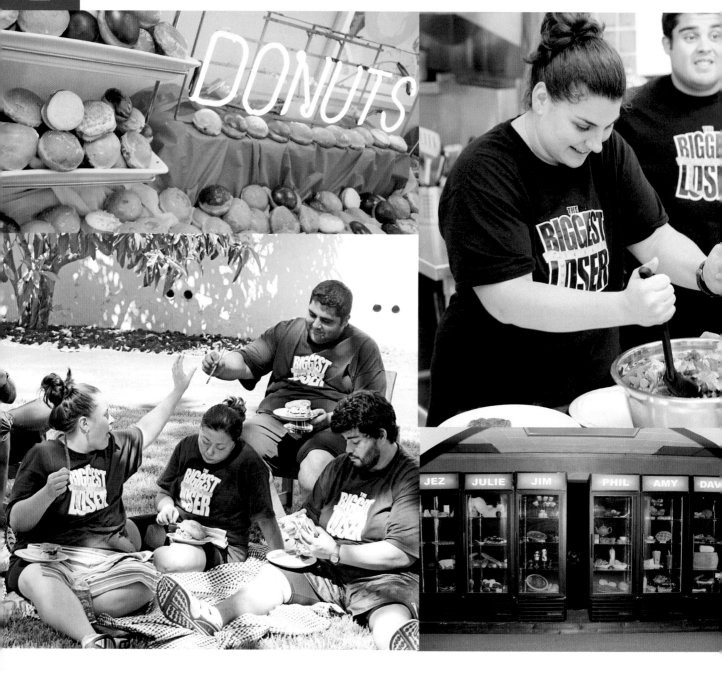

2

Eating Healthfully: Psychological Tips and Tricks

You've been watching *The Biggest Loser* and you're psyched up to start shedding pounds. You've already cleaned the junk food out of your pantry and refrigerator and stocked your kitchen with healthful foods. You're ready to change your I-don't-exercise ways. But hold on: Before your own amazing transformation can begin, consider some compelling research that shows it pays to have a few psychological tips and tricks up your sleeve to help you stay the course and make it to your goal weight.

Weight-loss researchers say that people who lose weight and keep it off don't just alter the way they eat and exercise. They modify their minds and behavior, too. Case in point: Researchers in Stockholm, Sweden, reviewed numerous studies to determine what helps

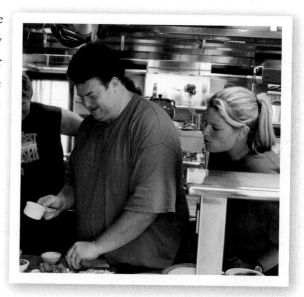

people shed weight and keep it off. According to their encouraging findings, published in the journal *Obesity Reviews*, successful weight loss is associated with a number of factors: leading a physically active lifestyle, adhering to a regular meal pattern that includes breakfast, eating healthfully, using reliable coping strategies to control overeating, and having psychological strength and stability.

In other words, changing the way you *think* about eating and exercising is just as important as changing your diet and exercise habits. The Biggest Losers have learned this principle, too—which is part of what makes them so successful at losing weight and keeping it off. Here are some of the strategies they've employed to get themselves into a successful weight-loss frame of mind.

Believe You Can Do It

Who doesn't remember the story of the Little Engine That Could? His memorable mantra—"I think I can"—was enough to help him climb even the steepest hills. Can your own self-talk help you do the same as you begin to lose weight?

The answer is a resounding yes. When you're on the road to your weight-loss goal, having a can-do attitude is key. And that attitude is controlled to a large extent by your faith in yourself and your ability to achieve your goals. In fact, your confidence needs to be even higher than the Little Engine's. He only thought he could. To be successful, you have to *know* you can.

Psychologists and motivational experts call this attitude *self-efficacy*. Put another way, it is believing in your ability to bring about a particular outcome. Unlike self-esteem, self-efficacy is specific to each situation or task that you face, such as exercising, eating healthfully, or controlling overeating. The stronger your self-efficacy becomes, the more resilient you are to setbacks and failure. If you truly believe in your ability to lose weight, then you can overcome the occasional setback by learning from it and moving on with even greater resolve.

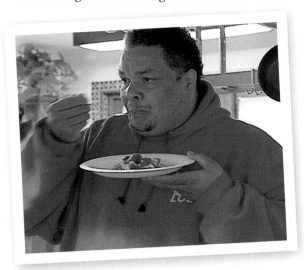

Pete Thomas, Season 2: "Success starts in the mind."

Pete Thomas from Season 2 has kept off 160 pounds, which is an amazing accomplishment. He says, "Believing that you can lose weight and keep it off is really vital. I do think that successful dieting and exercising start in the mind."

Learning from our mistakes so we don't make the same ones over and over again is also important. "The past is a great teacher," adds Pete. "Before you get started on your diet or exercise program, analyze which behaviors you did last time that worked for you—like getting up early to exercise or cutting back on sugary foods—and do them again. Use the success you had in the past for success now."

Don't Forget to Eat

Once you're in the right frame of mind—when you believe in your ability to lose weight—it's important to have a food plan in place. Without one, you leave yourself vulnerable to impulsive eating and old habits. Psychologically, a plan helps your mind stay organized, helping you avoid trouble and stay on track.

The Biggest Loser diet calls for three main meals a day, along with one or two snacks, according to Cheryl Forberg, RD, the show's nutritionist who helped design the diet. A lot of people who want to lose weight skip meals, thinking it will accelerate their weight loss. In actuality, this can lead to out-of-control hunger and overeating. Stick to a regular eating schedule to keep satiated and energized. That means breakfast *and* lunch and dinner, plus two snacks, every single day to keep your blood sugar stable. You're less likely to gain weight and more likely to lose when you divide your food into more frequent meals. If you go too long without food, your blood sugar will begin to drop and fatigue can set in. That's when you're most susceptible to binge eating and unhealthy cravings. Sticking to *The Biggest Loser* diet will prevent all this and keep your energy level high.

According to Forberg, each meal should contain a combination of carbs and protein, important for helping you feel full and keeping your energy high. Here's a sample day's menu: one egg with turkey bacon for breakfast; cherries, cottage cheese, and almonds for a midmorning snack; a spinach salad with skinless chicken breast and half

an apple for lunch; Greek-style plain, fat-free yogurt with blueberries for a midafternoon snack; and grilled salmon with steamed quinoa and broccoli and a peach for dinner.

The breakfasts you eat on *The Biggest Loser* diet are hearty and filling, and they keep you from late-morning "starvation eating." "I was always a big breakfast eater, and I was worried that breakfasts on *The Biggest Loser* diet would make me feel deprived," comments Jay Kruger, Season 5. "But they don't. With eggs or egg whites, Canadian-style bacon, and whole-wheat toast, you can have a satisfying breakfast. It's not like you're missing anything."

Sticking to a pattern of regular meals throughout the day also helps you take in the right number of calories, and *The Biggest Loser* diet plan is based on calorie control. Discounting fluctuations in fluid intake, when you consume more calories than you burn, you gain weight. When you burn more calories than you eat, you lose weight. Fat cells respond to this caloric deficit by breaking down their stored fat and releasing it into the bloodstream to be

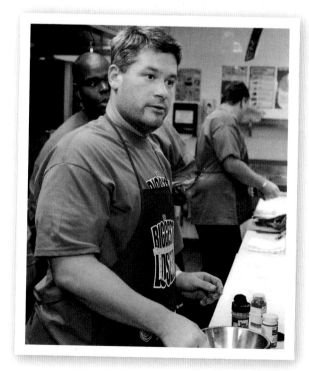

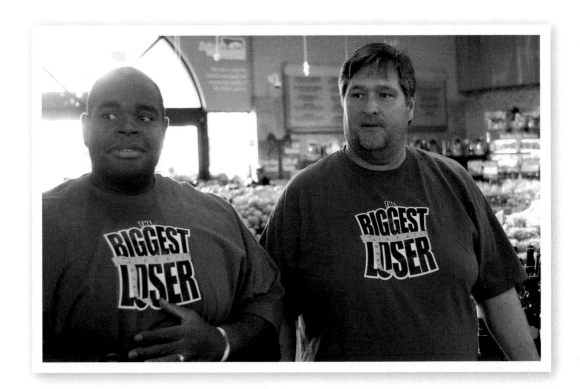

burned for energy. Every 3,500 unburned calories turn into 1 pound of fat, and every 3,500 burned calories convert into a pound lost. There is nothing bad or magical about calories; body weight just comes down to simple math. So you see, calories really do count when it comes to weight loss. And they count in another way, too: Structuring your eating plan around a calorie count helps to prevent spontaneous, uncontrolled eating.

Trent Patterson from Season 5 has a great system for organizing his daily calories: "I break them down to 500 for breakfast, 250 for my mid-day snack, 500 for lunch, 250 for my afternoon snack, and 500 for dinner. This method of planning my food has been very beneficial for me. I started out weighing 436 (I'm 6 feet tall), and in the first month, I lost 48 pounds. My clothes are already looser, and I can see the difference in the mirror. Calorie counting definitely works."

Trent's partner in Season 5, Roger Shultz, agrees. "Look at your calories as money. What do you want to spend them on? Would you spend several hundred on a soda that has all those empty calories and sugar, or would you rather spend them on a few bites of filet mignon? My budget is 2,000 calories a day. At first, I thought I'd starve, but I'm always satisfied and never feel deprived. Calorie counting helps control hunger pangs."

Can you deviate from your plan if you have room in your calorie budget to do so? Sure! In fact, it is OK to include your favorite foods from time to time, but in controlled portions. You can have the occasional cookie or slice of pizza—just don't eat a whole package of Oreos or an entire pizza pie in one sitting.

Write Down Everything You Eat

One of the most effective weight-control practices you can adopt is keeping a journal. Keep an uncensored food and exercise journal throughout your weight-loss journey, including all the details you would if you were pouring your heart out to your best friend. This includes writing down everything you eat, good or bad, along with how much of what kinds of exercise you do. You might even want to write down how you feel after eating different foods, so you'll have a record of what works for you and what doesn't. For example, if eating an apple didn't satisfy your sugar craving but a sugar-free Popsicle did the trick, write that down. You'll have a winning strategy ready the next time your sweet tooth calls. Keeping a journal increases opportunities for weight-loss success. In fact,

research shows that dieters who record what they consume every day drop twice as much weight as those who don't.

Isabeau Miller, Season 4: "A food journal keeps you honest."

Every season, the contestants are required to show their food journals to their trainers and to one of the show's physicians, Dr. Robert Huizenga. "This is an important monitoring tool that helps them stay the course, " he says. Season 4 finalist Isabeau Miller says it works for her. "Writing down what I eat keeps me honest, and within my calorie

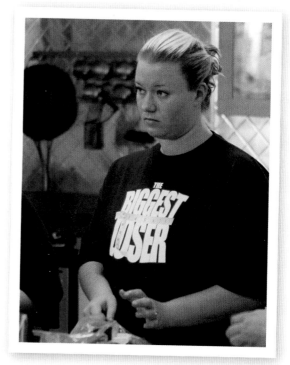

range. I realize I don't have to cut everything I love out of my diet, like ice cream. I can have a small scoop, as long as I stay within my daily calorie allowance. Seeing my eating habits on paper helps keep me accountable for every morsel, too. And if the needle on the scale doesn't move, all I have to do is look at my journal to see what I ate."

Kelly MacFarland from Season 1 says that she keeps a food journal to this day, and she credits it with helping her keep off 65 of the 72 pounds she lost at the ranch. "My food journal helps me plan my meals, and I'm less likely to deviate. I write everything down, even if it's not pretty."

Keeping a food journal is clearly an effective method for tracking your food intake. It's personalized, adaptable, and as detailed as you want to make it. As you lose pounds, you'll gain something else: insight into when and why you overeat. Don't be surprised if you learn that you're feeding your stomach when you really should be feeding your soul.

Pete Thomas, Season 2: "Analyze your day."

Pete Thomas, Season 2's winner of the eliminated players, analyzes his journal at the end of every day and grades himself on how he did. "I ask myself: What can I do better tomorrow? What do I need to change? And I make adjustments." By analyzing your journal, you'll not only learn about your eating habits, you'll also discover the unique aspects of your journey toward health. You'll see the patterns of your life unfold, you'll reclaim who you really are, and you'll continue to achieve your goals.

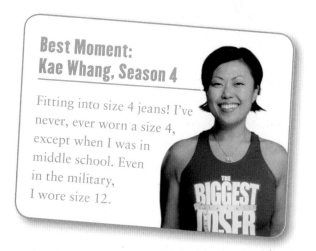

Best Moment: Kae Whang, Season 4

Fitting into size 4 jeans! I've never, ever worn a size 4, except when I was in middle school. Even in the military, I wore size 12.

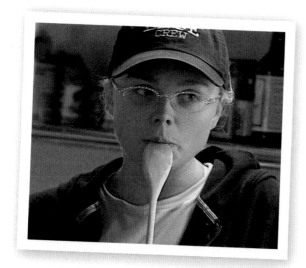

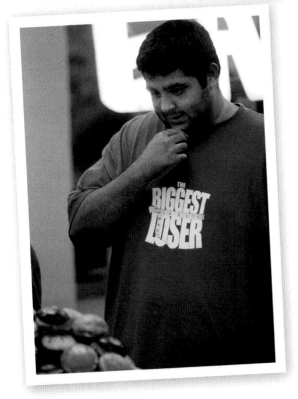

Learn New Cooking Techniques

At the heart of *The Biggest Loser* program is food—plenty of it, put together in a plan that is easy, healthful, enjoyable to follow, and designed to help you shed pounds. When you are trying to lose weight and have a lot of it to lose, you want to make sure your food is tasty. The more adventurous you are with your food choices and preparation, the less bored you'll be with your diet.

"I've learned how to turn any fattening dish into something low cal and healthy—and no one can tell the difference," says Season 2 finalist Suzy Preston. "For example, I make lasagna with lean ground beef and low-fat cottage cheese—and I substitute zucchini strips for the lasagna noodles. My mashed potatoes are a combination of potatoes, mashed cauliflower, and fat-free milk—they're delicious, and everyone thinks they're the 'real thing.'"

Neil Tejwani, Season 4, has learned the same techniques. "Let's say you want a grilled cheese sandwich. Prepare your sandwich using low-fat cheese, no-calorie butter spray, and two slices of high-fiber bread. You can put the sandwich in a toaster oven as an easy and low-fat alternative to frying it. This type of recipe still satisfies your craving, yet you're only eating a third of the calories you normally would if you were eating a full-fat, high-calorie sandwich."

Take a cue from Suzy and Neil and have fun

The Biggest Losers Weigh In on Holiday and Party Temptations

Food temptations are everywhere during the holidays. Office parties, tins packed with homemade cookies, and festive cocktails offer little escape. Here's what the Biggest Losers advise to help you enjoy the holidays and still keep your program intact.

Hollie Self, Season 4:

If the holiday meal is a special one for you, plan to enjoy it. Make an agreement with yourself that it is okay to not have a weight-loss day. You've worked hard thus far and enjoying a holiday dinner is not going to ruin anything. And keep your indulgences to just the meal, not the entire holiday.

Kelly MacFarland, Season 1:

Don't beat yourself up if you go out for drinks and dinner with your friends and overindulge. Get up the next morning knowing that it's a new day and a renewed chance to live an active, healthy life. Find some balance on a daily basis, so when you do have those indulgences, it's not a big deal and you can work through them. You always have the gym and your sneakers, so if you feel like you've blown it, then you just have to work it off, and there is no guilt.

Pam Smith, Season 3:

Don't go to the party or holiday meal famished. Being too hungry will set you up for gorging. Focus on those foods that you love, eat slowly, and give yourself permission to savor them. Another strategy is to bring some of your own healthy food to share.

Suzy Preston, Season 2:

Try to arrange activities with your friends that don't include food, such as going to the movies, a concert, or a play—or do something active together, like skiing or ice-skating. This strategy works all the time, not just around the holidays.

Kae Whang, Season 4:

The holiday season is a time to celebrate good times with family and friends. Try to make the focus more on socializing and less on eating. Listen to your body, too. It will say, "I'm full." So don't have seconds or thirds. The goal is to have a great time and enjoy your company.

Kelly Fields, Season 5:

I like to have a happy hour about once a week. But I used to drink Long Island iced teas, which are highly caloric. If you want to drink at a holiday party, have some light beer or a couple of tequila shots, and do it responsibly. When the holidays come around, it's all about doing things a little bit smarter.

experimenting. Spice up your foods with herbs, salsa, seasonings, artificial sweeteners, salt substitutes, vinegars, mustard, low-sodium ketchup, hot sauce, chili paste, and so forth. Or explore the local farmers' market for something exotic like bok choy, or sprinkle new spices on your staple meals. (Chili powder is a favorite in *The Biggest Loser* kitchen.) And learn new light-cooking techniques. Thumb through *The Biggest Loser Cookbook* or browse through recipes online for some healthy tricks and then modify a favorite high-fat dish.

Handle Cravings Sensibly

Many people who are trying to lose weight struggle with cravings, bingeing, and nighttime refrigerator raids—and the Biggest Losers are no exceptions. At some point, all of them have expe-

rienced a hankering for chocolate or chips and dip or a big bowl of macaroni and cheese.

There's a big difference between cravings and hunger pangs, though. When you're hungry, you'll usually eat anything. Cravings are more specific. You crave a certain type of food that fufills a specific taste or need. Cravings also tend to occur at particular times and in particular situations, like during the midafternoon, when your blood sugar typically plummets and you feel sluggish and in need of a lift; when you're stressed out or bored; the days right before your menstrual period, if you're a woman; or when you see something tempting, like a fast-food commercial on TV. All of these things give rise to cravings, but that can be a good thing, because forewarned is forearmed: If you know when and where a food craving is going to strike, you can avoid it.

Too often people skip breakfast or forget about lunch, only to feel a craving strike later in the day. Think ahead and plan a healthful breakfast, lunch, and dinner that consist of carbohydrates, protein, and good fats. Eat carbs, protein, and a little fat with every meal and snack. When you eat meals that are lacking in one kind of nutrient, you may be more likely to crave it later. Protein and fat take longer to digest than carbs, so include them, along with more fiber, in every meal to help you feel satisfied longer. Says Season 1's Kelly MacFarland,

BIGGEST LOSER TOOLBOX

"In addition to a structured exercise routine, try to put more 'lifestyle activity' into your day. This could mean walking down the street to talk to a neighbor or even just taking the stairs instead of the elevator at work. It's an easy way to zap some extra calories."

—Bill Germanakos, Season 4 winner

"If my meals are monotonous—the same day after day—I sometimes experience powerful cravings."

David Griffin, Season 4: "Avoid binge foods until you can handle them."

Although it's okay to sample your favorite foods every now and then, it's wise to avoid foods that still tempt you to binge. So if you can't handle eating only a small quantity of your favorite foods, stay away from them for now. This is a tactic used by David Griffin, who admits to having an addictive personality when it comes to food. "If I allow myself a treat every day or every other day, then

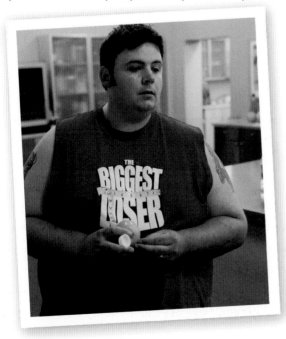

BIGGEST LOSER TOOLBOX

"Don't eat food out of its original container. You'll eat more than you think. Measure out your portion and place it on a plate."

—Trent Patterson, Season 5

I'm going to be eating it two to three times a day again. To keep cravings at bay, I choose low-calorie alternatives, such as fat-free pudding or sugar-free Popsicles. These give me the feeling of having an indulgence without indulging."

One of the craving-control techniques employed by the Biggest Losers is walking away from temptations. If you really crave a food, walk away from it for 15 minutes and do something that's not food-related to keep your mind busy. If you still want it after 15 minutes, then eat it. "You don't need to deprive yourself of anything," says Jenn Widder, Season 5, who uses this tactic. "Just don't binge and go overboard. This is a strategy you can use for the rest of your life."

Jenn's partner in Season 5, Maggie King, agrees: "I've learned that if I feel a craving coming on, I should substitute eating with a nonfood activity, such as getting a manicure or pedicure. Do something nice for yourself. It will take your mind off food."

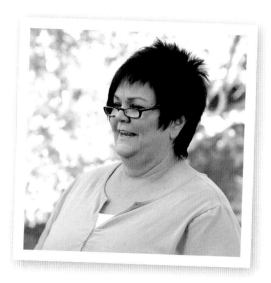

Bette-Sue Burklund, Season 5: "Substitute fruit for candy if you have a sweet tooth."

What about cravings for sweets like candy, cake, or ice cream? How do you keep them in check, especially if you have a sweet tooth? Eating sweets might increase the brain's level of serotonin, a feel-good chemical that raises your spirits—so your cravings for sweets might actually be symptoms of a desire for an emotional lift. To get the same feeling, you could reach for healthful carbs such as whole-grain bread or a baked sweet potato, or exercise to elevate your mood. If you still feel a craving for something sweet, do what Bette-Sue Burkland does when she gets an urge for candy. "I substitute fruit," she says. "Instead of a box of sour candy, for example, I eat a tangerine." The fiber in fruit helps slow sugar absorption. This prevents fluctuations in your blood sugar so you don't get more cravings later.

Another strategy taught on *The Biggest Loser* set is to ask yourself if giving in to a craving is worth it. Kae Whang, Season 4, elaborates: "Is it worth knowing that you have to work out the next day? If the answer is yes, I go for it. If the answer is no, I don't eat it. The 'Is it worth it?' motto has really stuck with me."

Behind the scenes on *The Biggest Loser*, cast members are allowed to have one "high-calorie day" a week, if they so choose. This doesn't mean that they indulge in a caloric free-for-all, but they can include foods not normally in their diet as long as they count them toward their daily calorie allot-

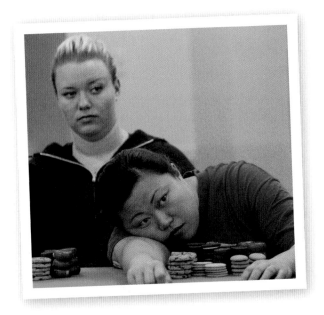

ment. Explains Season 4's Jim Germanakos, "Some of us called these foods 'cheat foods,' and others called them 'birthday presents.' It's okay to eat them; you just have to be very careful to work the calories into your calorie count. For me, this was a lifesaver. When I was craving things like pizza and ice cream, having a high-calorie day didn't make me feel like I could never eat these things again. It made me feel like there was a time and place for these foods, in moderation."

Tame Your Temptations

You've seen those episodes of *The Biggest Loser* in which the contestants are faced with the choice of consuming mounds of pudding or towers of doughnuts in exchange for cash or some equally alluring payoff. In reality, contestants are faced with such foods every day they're at the ranch. Temptations are kept around at all times. You might think that's cruel, but it makes sense. The Biggest Losers will have access to all that stuff in the real world—so they have got to learn how to resist temptations.

The more we deprive ourselves of certain foods, the more we tend to think about them. Denying yourself backfires. If you say you're never going to eat chocolate again, chocolate instantly becomes the thing you most crave, and you may spend an inordinate amount of time daydreaming

about it. Before long, you'll be biting down on a candy bar . . . or two or three.

No food should be categorically forbidden. The trick is to find the right balance, to let yourself have a planned treat in a small quantity every now and again without letting it turn into a binge. Find your happy medium.

There's really nothing you can't eat; you just can't eat it in excess, or you have to burn off an equivalent caloric amount with exercise. "One of my favorite foods, for example, is cheese puffs," says Ali Vincent from Season 5. "I can still have them. I just have to make sure they're in my calorie budget—or that I burn them off with exercise. Whatever you put in your mouth, you've got to make sure you burn off, too."

As Ali suggests, if you properly manage your calories, you can eat a tempting food if you want it. "One time we had a temptation challenge in which doughnuts were put in front of us," recalls Season 4 winner Bill Germanakos. "We all

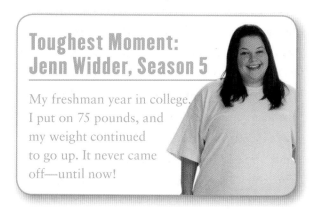

Toughest Moment: Jenn Widder, Season 5

My freshman year in college, I put on 75 pounds, and my weight continued to go up. It never came off—until now!

The Biggest Loser Online Club Profile: **Jeremy Grey**

Starting weight: 400 • Current weight: 228 • Goal weight: 200

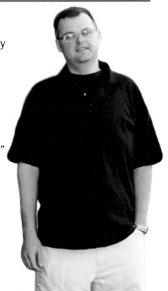

For Jeremy, joining *The Biggest Loser* Online Club was about learning how to eat healthy again. "We used to go out to eat on a regular basis. Basically, I would eat whatever I wanted and as much as I wanted. After I joined, I realized that that wasn't an option."

What Jeremy likes most about the Club is that it makes things simple for you. "All the guesswork is gone: The fully customizable menu is there for you, the calories are laid out for you, the workout routines are created for you, and it tracks your progress."

Now that his body is used to healthy food, he wishes he had eaten this way from the start. "I have told people time and time again, 'If I knew as a teenager what I know now, I would have never gained the weight in the first place.'"

Jeremy's advice to others is to not give up. "You can do it! Losing weight and becoming healthy is one of the best things you can do to show your family you love them and care about them."

Change your life today! Log on to www.biggestloserclub.com and get started.

budgeted a few extra calories so that we could eat a few doughnuts. I ate three and was lucky enough to find the gold coin that was worth $5,000!"

Look at Healthy Foods in a New Light

The Biggest Loser nutritionist Cheryl Forberg, RD, cautions that when you're trying to take off pounds: "Just say 'no' to the white stuff—pasta, sugar, and flour." The Biggest Losers who have lost weight and kept it off changed the way they view food. They

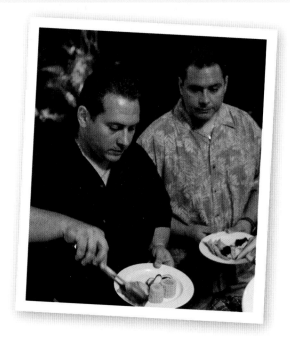

10 Easy Low-Cal Desserts

1. **Ricotta Fruit Cup.** Fill a wineglass or parfait glass half-full with blueberries or fresh sliced strawberries. Top with ½ cup fat-free ricotta cheese, then drizzle with honey and sprinkle with cinnamon.

2. **Roasted Fruits with Honey.** Halve fruits such as peaches or nectarines and remove the pits. Place on a baking sheet and drizzle each half with 1 teaspoon honey. Roast in a 350°F oven until tender and juicy, about 15 minutes.

3. **Banana–Peanut Butter Sandwich.** Peel a banana and cut it in half lengthwise. Spread 1 tablespoon creamy reduced-fat peanut butter onto the cut side of one half, then top with the other half to create a banana sandwich. Cut into bite-size pieces, if desired.

4. **Low-Cal "Ice Cream" Sandwich.** Create a homemade frozen treat by sandwiching 2 tablespoons sugar-free whipped topping between 2 fat-free chocolate graham crackers. Cover with plastic wrap and pop into the freezer for 1 hour.

5. **Baked Maple Apple.** Core and halve an unpeeled apple and place it in a small microwavable bowl. Cover with plastic wrap and heat on high power in a microwave for 2 minutes. Drizzle each half with 1 tablespoon sugar-free maple syrup, then sprinkle with cinnamon or allspice.

6. **Low-Cal Peanut Butter Cup.** Stir 1 teaspoon creamy reduced-fat peanut butter into a sugar-free, fat-free chocolate pudding cup. It tastes just like a peanut butter cup!

7. **Banana Milkshake.** Peel an extra-ripe banana, cut it into chunks, and freeze in a ziptop bag. In a blender, process the frozen chunks with 1 cup fat-free milk or fat-free yogurt.

8. **Healthy Latte.** For a healthier alternative to the drinks sold at many coffee chains, pour 1 cup of cooled coffee over ice, add a small scoop of fat-free vanilla frozen yogurt, and top with a sprinkling of nutmeg or cocoa powder.

9. **Angel Food Trifle.** In a parfait glass, layer 2 small chunks of angel food cake (equal to one slice) with sliced berries of your choice and ½ cup fat-free frozen yogurt.

10. **Not-So-Decadent Chocolate-Covered Strawberries.** Dip 5 or 6 large fresh strawberries into 2 tablespoons fat-free chocolate sauce for a guilt-free version of chocolate-covered strawberries.

educated themselves about good nutrition and made a commitment to enjoying healthful, lower-fat foods. They did this by focusing on the positive aspect of what they were eating—viewing healthful foods as desirable foods that fuel and nourish their bodies. In other words, they adopted a new "food attitude."

Along the way, their palates actually changed, and they found themselves enjoying—and desiring—healthier choices. Says Isabeau Miller, Season 4 finalist: "You can actually train your body to want healthier foods. That's what happened to me. I now find myself craving fresh fruit, fresh vegetables, and organic meat."

Face Emotional Eating Head On

"I was so bored, I ate a whole bag of chips." "My husband and I had a fight and I headed straight for the refrigerator." "I eat really healthy, but whenever I'm at my in-laws', I go hog wild."

Can you relate to these situations? Are you likely to eat for all the wrong reasons? Emotions—either positive or negative—can drive us toward food for comfort or escape. Whether we're dealing with loneliness, anxiety, depression, boredom, or even joy, many of us reach for food. Because eating feels good, most people (fat and thin alike) end up using food as a ready source of emotional release or a way to ease stress and anxiety. When our emotions are triggered, it provokes a psychological hunger, and we can eat a lot of food in a short period of time.

How we think can also influence how much we eat. Certain thoughts may give you trouble—for example, believing that your diet is an all-or-nothing matter, that if you eat some forbidden food or skip an exercise class, all your efforts are for nothing. It's this kind of thinking, not the act of slipping up, that can make you feel like a failure and weaken your resolve to stick with your program. It is unrealistic to think that you can eat a perfect diet all the time. If you expect perfection from yourself, you really are setting yourself up for failure. Changing this mind-set and adopting a more moderate approach can help you lose weight and keep it off.

Once you learn more dependable ways to deal with eating-related emotions, you can leave emotional eating behind for good and move forward

BIGGEST LOSER TOOLBOX

"Enjoy a salad or some broth-based soup prior to your entrée when eating out. You'll feel full before you get to your entrée, and you're less likely to overeat."
—Matt Hoover, Season 2 winner

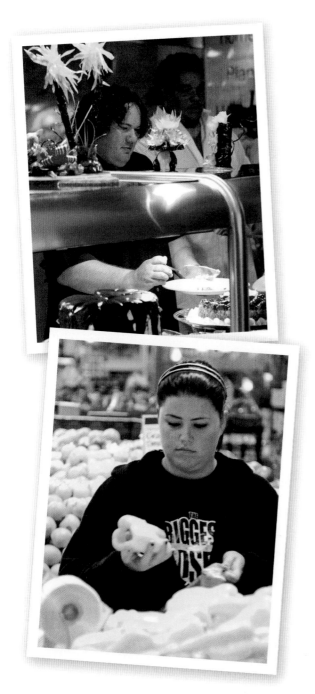

with alternative coping skills. All the contestants had to explore their relationships with food, stop allowing their moods to determine what and how much they ate, and learn how to take control of their eating. A powerful example of this is Matt Hoover, who took home $250,000 for being the Biggest Loser in Season 2.

"I admit, I'm an emotional eater. In the past, I let myself believe things like 'Oh, I'm no good; I'm the happy, fat, drunk guy.' I played it up great," Matt says. "No one knew I was depressed, but at night when I'd go home, I didn't turn on the lights. I didn't want to see what I looked like. I didn't turn on the lights in the morning when I was getting dressed because I was trying to tuck in my shirt and suck in my breath and button my pants and tie my shoes. It was uncomfortable. I just accepted that way of living."

Then Matt got on the show and started seeing his body and his health change. As these changes occurred, he realized that he had been selling himself short. "I gained my weight because I felt bad. I kept my weight because I felt bad, but as I started feeling better, I started losing that. I started losing the weight and the bad anger and the hurt. As you start caring about yourself more, your weight will start coming off."

Brittany Aberle, age 22, Season 5, confesses to being a lifelong emotional eater. Her parents

"If you know the evening is when you usually overindulge, save your calories for that time. Make them work for you and don't fight it all day. I save up for the evening and have air-popped popcorn with low-cal butter spray. I always have precut veggies ready for my 'snacky' moments."

—Suzy Preston, Season 2 finalist

divorced when she was 7, and she blamed herself. By the time she was 8, she was overweight and remained that way ever since. "Most people I know think this is the best time of their lives, but for me, it's been one of the worst," she says.

Brittany just ended a 6-year relationship that had deteriorated in the last few years. Her boyfriend was very critical of her weight, and it was a huge problem. "The more he criticized me, the more I ate," she says.

When she arrived at *The Biggest Loser* ranch, she weighed 221 pounds. Happily, she shed 18 pounds in the first 3 weeks. "After being there just a short time and learning the principles of lifestyle change, I began to get my emotional eating under control. For one thing, I learned that food is for fuel and nourishment. It's not something to medicate negative emotions away. Eating five small meals a day of healthy foods has established a pat-

tern that satisfies my need for nourishment. When I feel tense, I know I can do things like exercise or yoga to release the tension. I realize that I am going to have a happy life and that I'm going to get my weight under control. It's not going to be a lifelong problem anymore."

Isabeau Miller, Season 4: "Keep yourself busy."

When you feel stressed, down in the dumps, angry, bored, or another emotion that prompts you to eat, do something on your list of "go to" activities, such as taking your dog for a walk, roller-skating, painting—anything that will keep your mind occu-

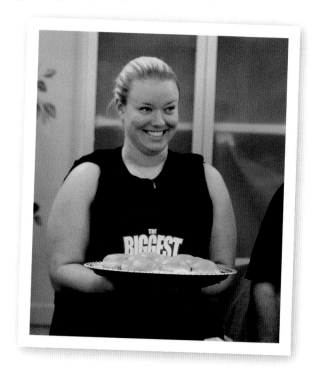

pied. That way, you won't fill up unstructured time with food.

"Redirect your activity and do something different," says Isabeau Miller, a Season 4 finalist. "For example, rather than staying home by yourself and risking feeling lonely, call a friend and invite him or her out to a movie or another activity, or simply call friends and talk on the phone. Have a more structured schedule to prevent boredom."

Kae Whang, Season 4, suggests learning yoga or meditation to prevent emotional eating when a bad mood strikes. "Besides being a distraction, these activities have a calming effect on your body, mind, and spirit." Yoga and meditation have also been proven to help your mind focus more sharply.

At *The Biggest Loser* ranch, contestants spend a lot of time digging down deep to find out why they eat emotionally. You, too, have to learn to deal directly with what upsets you, and this may require the help of a qualified therapist. Once you acknowledge what the problem is, you can start to change it.

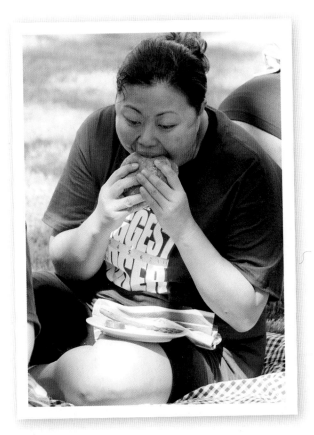

There you have it—real-life, real-world success strategies for sticking to your nutrition plan and shedding pounds in the process. Once you start following advice from the Biggest Losers (there's lots more to come), you're setting yourself up for success. They did it—and so can you!

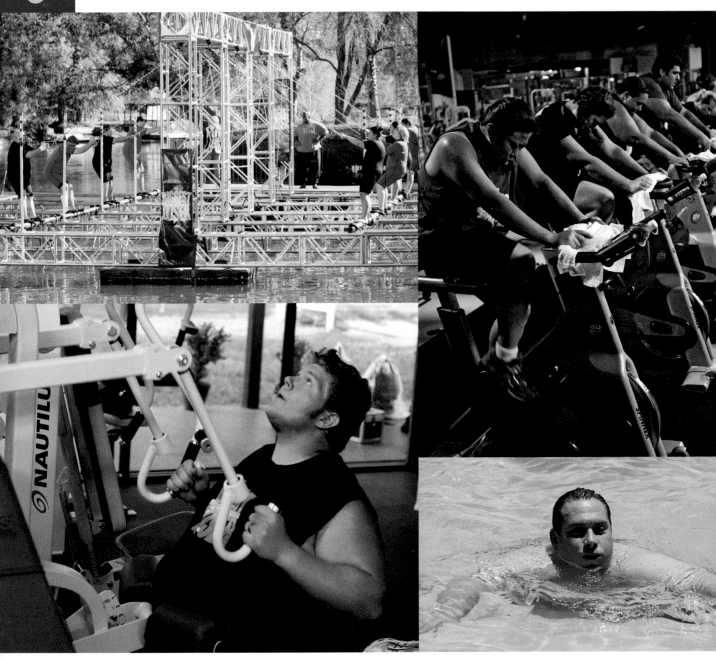

3

Burning Calories: Motivation to Get Moving and Keep Moving

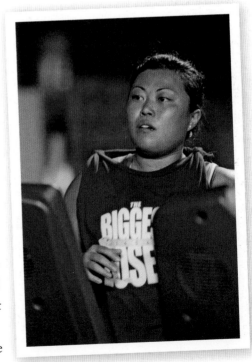

People who successfully lose weight have one thing in common: exercise. In fact, research shows most of them burn 2,500 or more extra calories a week through exercise. That's the weekly equivalent of 75 minutes of brisk walking (or alternating walking with 60 minutes of vigorous circuit training) each day—pretty doable by most standards. So why aren't more of us doing it?

It takes consistency and determination to make exercise a habit. Sure, we all get excited by the idea of being fit and athletic, but often we don't follow through on the daily commitment required to actually get off our duffs and do something. There's a reason why health clubs are packed in January and empty in March—making the resolution is easy, but making it a habit is tough.

If you want to get motivated and stay motivated, you've

come to the right place. This is the chapter where you'll find fitness guidance from the Biggest Losers, many of whom have forged consistent, successful workout programs, lost hundreds of pounds, and stayed trim and fit in the process.

Excuse-Proof Your Exercise Program

It's easy to find an excuse not to exercise: "I'm too fat." "It hurts my knees." "I have diabetes." "I don't like exercise." "I can't afford it." But keep in mind that if you want to construct a stronger, sexier body, boost your energy, feel invigorated, and gain other impressive payoffs, you've got to stop making excuses for not changing a couch-potato lifestyle.

One of the best ways to ensure that you'll stick with your exercise plan is to find activities you love and can incorporate into your life. After all, exercise should be fun. Having a good time while you're exercising will produce better results, because you'll be more likely to stick to a plan you enjoy.

Kae Whang, Season 4, adds, "I've fallen in love with boxing—it is very empowering—and I'm hoping to enter a boxing tournament next year. I also enjoy rock climbing. It's great for your arms! Another suggestion I have: charity runs. They're fun, and you can walk or run to support causes you're passionate about."

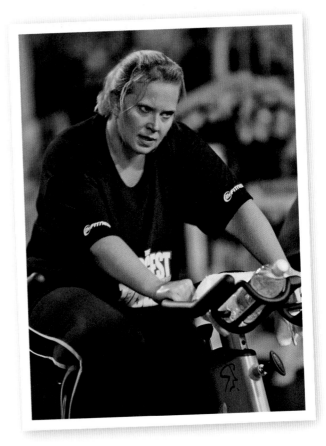

While exercise should always be challenging, it's also important to choose exercises that you're comfortable with and that suit your body's strengths. For example, if you are proud of your strong arms, you might want to give rowing a try. If you know that your core muscles are your best assets, Pilates could be a great fit for you. How efficiently or expertly you do anything, from running a mile to doing a spin class, will enhance your interest in doing it—not to mention your results. "Your motivation multiplies when you know you can be successful. However, don't give up too easily as you experiment with different activities," urges Julie Hadden, Season 4 runner-up.

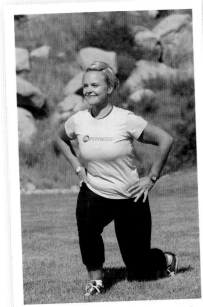

Even if it's an activity you like, exercising is hard work, and it can be easy to talk yourself into quitting. Working with a personal trainer, at least occasionally, can help you avoid this sort of negative attitude. Says Pam Smith, Season 3, "I believe that when you're overweight and struggling to stay active, you need someone to encourage you to stay in the game."

"If you can't enlist the services of a personal trainer, consider having an exercise partner to keep you motivated," advises Suzy Preston, Season 2 runner-up. "When I was on the ranch, I'd run with Seth, a friend on the men's team. He would push me by saying, 'Don't hold on to the treadmill,' and I'd say back, 'Okay, crank it up then.' This experience taught me the value of having a training

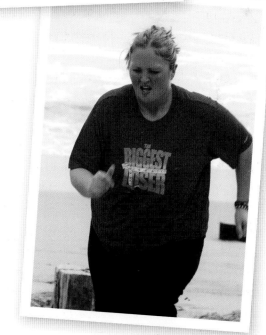

partner. These days, I work out with a friend first thing in the morning. We do weight training 2 days a week and cardio 5 or 6 days a week. We do something different every time, too—a must for me since I'm easily bored."

Having a workout partner also keeps you accountable. After all, you're less likely to duck out of an exercise appointment if your partner is counting on you to be there. Another idea is to join

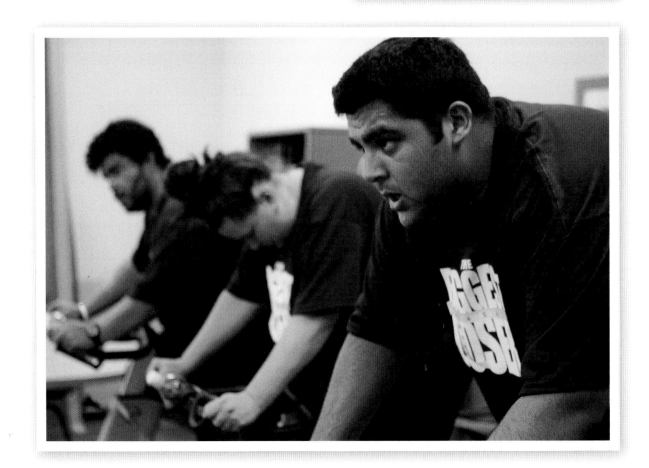

a class or sports league where people count on you to show up. If your basketball team or dance partner depends on you, you will not want to let them down by missing a class or game.

Sometimes the hardest part of going to the gym is just getting in the door. Once you're there, even if you're doing something low impact, it's still better than sitting at home. Psych yourself up by focusing on all of the powerful benefits of exercise, from losing fat, to building strength, to boosting your immune system. Neil Tejwani, Season 4, says, "If you work out even 30 minutes a day for 4 or 5 days a week, that can potentially make you healthier. That's the way I look at it now: I'm sacrificing 30 minutes a day to potentially add years to my life."

"If you could bottle the benefits of exercise—which boosts your energy, bolsters your immune system, lifts depression, protects you from heart attacks, and even extends your active years—it would be the most prescribed medication in the world," says Dr. Robert Huizenga, one of the show's medical consultants. There are piles of proof that exercise has more overall impact on your health than any other health-related action you can take. In fact, one landmark study found that those whose only health risk was inactivity were more apt to die prematurely than daily exercisers with high cholesterol and high blood pressure. In other words, sitting around, day in and day out, is hazardous to your health.

Merely understanding the effects of exercise on your body isn't always enough to get you moving. Try to personalize the benefits. For example, you know that cardio training is great for your heart. Okay, what does that mean to you? Better results on your physicals, year after year? Greater protection against heart disease, which runs in your family? Personalizing the rewards of exercise can make all the difference on your journey to better health and fitness.

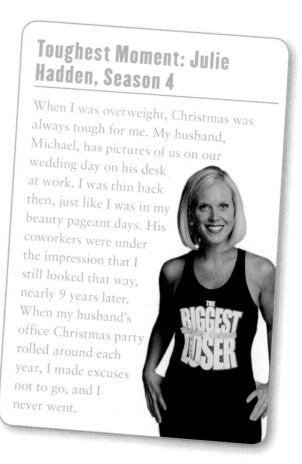

Toughest Moment: Julie Hadden, Season 4

When I was overweight, Christmas was always tough for me. My husband, Michael, has pictures of us on our wedding day on his desk at work. I was thin back then, just like I was in my beauty pageant days. His coworkers were under the impression that I still looked that way, nearly 9 years later. When my husband's office Christmas party rolled around each year, I made excuses not to go, and I never went.

Some people use the excuse that they can't afford to work out. After all, exercise can be pricey, depending on where you work out and what type of equipment you need. But there are many budget-friendly and effective exercises you can do that don't require monthly membership fees. Resistance bands, stability balls, and free weights are all low-cost and effective alternatives to more expensive equipment. You don't need heavy weights, either. If performed properly, high-repetition resistance exercises using light to moderately heavy weights can actually burn more calories than doing fewer reps with more weight. You can also take advantage of ordinary things around the house—climb the stairs for 5 to 10 minutes, do crunches, or try pushups on your knees.

"Sidewalks are completely free," says Matt Hoover, Season 2's winner. "Just get out there and walk. Start with 1 block, then add 2 blocks, and build toward doing a mile or more."

Paul Marks from Season 5 adds this tip: "Another great exercise tool is furry and has four legs—your dog! Take your dog out for brisk walks to fit in some exercise. You can really elevate your heart rate and burn fat. Your dog will be happy, too, since pets love being active. I have two shelties, and they look forward to their walks with me every day. For someone who is timid about going to the gym or can't afford it, this option is terrific."

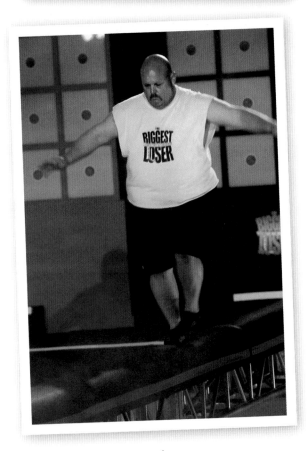

Burn the Calories, Lose the Fat

You've heard it a thousand times: Movement is vital for losing weight. Exercise burns excess calories that would otherwise be stored as fat. When combined with a sensible nutrition program, regular exercise also may elevate the metabolic rate, and in just the right setting, promote muscle growth. During a calorie-restricted diet, exercise helps preserve muscle to keep your metabolism high. But when you diet without exercising, your body may use up muscle, causing your metabolism to slow down. You won't get all the body-firming benefits of exercise. While you don't have to replicate every *Biggest Loser* workout you've seen on TV, you do have to get your body moving at some level of effort and intensity.

Julie Hadden, Season 4's runner-up, emphasizes that it is important to challenge yourself to get the weight-loss results you want. "If your routine feels comfortable, devote a few more minutes

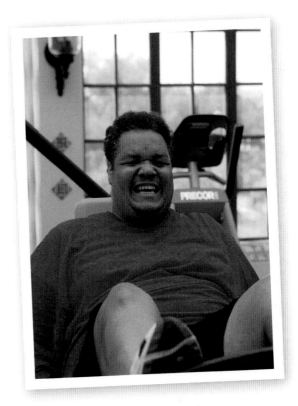

to each workout, or add hills and/or stairs to your regular walk. Do more to achieve more. After every workout, congratulate yourself on having accomplished something and taking another step toward your goal."

You've probably seen some novel but intense ways of working out on *The Biggest Loser*, some of which can easily be integrated into your own workout at home. One of these workout ideas is the "push cart," performed on a treadmill with the electricity turned off. This move is a favorite of

---

BIGGEST LOSER TOOLBOX

"Do your weight training prior to your cardio session. It will help you to burn more fat while you do cardio."
—Jim Germanakos, Season 4

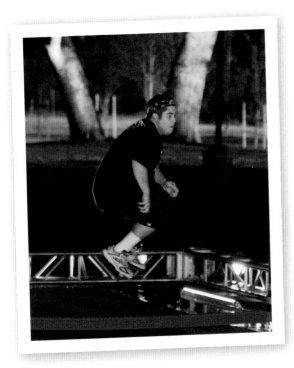

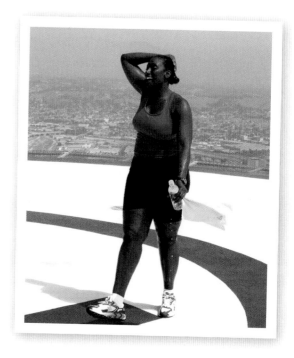

Bernie Salazar's from Season 5. "You walk on the treadmill, making the belt move under your own power. It's an amazing workout! If you don't have a treadmill or think you can't afford one, shop around at garage sales and look for a broken one on which you can do this really cool—and challenging—exercise."

A lot of viewers might get the impression that they have to work out for 4 or more hours a day like the contestants do on the show. Not true. But you do have to be intense. Explains Kae Whang, Season 4: "I have a trainer at home who puts me through 30-minute workouts that are so intense that sometimes I feel like I just want to fall over. If you put 110 percent into a single 30-minute workout, you're going to get more results than if you exercised for an hour at 80 percent effort."

Once they get to the ranch, most contestants

BIGGEST LOSER TOOLBOX

"Make sure you sweat. You need to challenge yourself to get the results you want. If your routine feels comfortable, devote a few more minutes to each workout, or add hills to your regular walk."

—Isabeau Miller, Season 4 finalist

find out fast how out of shape they are, and this often has a motivating effect. "Right after we got to the ranch, we were put through the Presidential Fitness Test, and I couldn't do a pullup," says Mark Kruger, Season 5. "It bothered me like nobody's business, so I set a goal to build my upper-body strength. I'm going to work as hard as I can to get to that goal. It's very important to have exercise goals like that—something to look forward to, something to motivate you."

What about after they leave the ranch? How do contestants stick with their exercise routines? Pete Thomas, who has done a remarkable job of staying trim and buff since Season 2, has this to

Best Moment: Jackie Evans, Season 5

In Season 5, we all had "goal flags" to keep us motivated. My flag said, "Put on my wedding ring." I've been married for 31 years, which I'm very proud of, but my wedding ring didn't fit on my finger anymore. I was too fat. Within 3 weeks of being on *The Biggest Loser* and losing 30 pounds, I was able to put my wedding ring on. That was the best moment of all.

BIGGEST LOSER TOOLBOX

"Work out to your favorite music. It's motivating and makes your workout go by in a flash."

—Erik Chopin, Season 3 winner

say: "When I was on *The Biggest Loser*, I looked at it as my last chance. I had to get it right! Once I left the ranch, I was determined to take what I had learned and apply it to real life. Some statistics say that people lose weight but gain it back within 5 years, so I set a 5-year goal for myself to maintain my exercise and nutrition habits. From there, I set mini-goals. For instance, on a daily basis, I keep a log and I take a few minutes to review how I'm doing. I look for patterns in my behavior. If I had a busy travel week, for example, and didn't make it to the gym, that tells me that next time, I should pack my running shoes. You can't approach exercise as something you do just to get in shape for bathing suit season or a high school reunion. Working out and staying fit is a lifetime endeavor, and we all need to be in it for the long haul."

One of the best moves for taking weight off and keeping it off is to incorporate strength training into your workout. It boosts your metabolism and increases the amount of calorie-burning muscle on your frame. Work each muscle group at least twice a week, with 2 days off in between. For

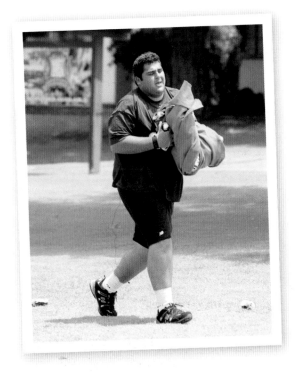

many people, that translates into 20 minutes 4 days a week—2 days for the upper body and 2 days for the lower body. "I came to *The Biggest Loser* wanting to pull my own weight, and I did that— both literally and figuratively," says Isabeau Miller, Season 4 finalist. "I've noticed changes in my body so much more quickly since I started weight training, and now I can lift as much as the guys can."

Maybe you saw *The Biggest Loser* episode in Season 4 in which the cast members were presented with their "before" pictures. Most cast members now use those photos as a tool to maintain the intensity, to keep them from returning to their former fat selves.

"I have a picture on my mirror of the old Neil,

The Biggest Loser Online Club Profile: Rommy Engel

Starting weight: 167 • Current weight: 136

Rommy is close to achieving a lifelong dream: running a full marathon. After competing in several half-marathons, she's hoping to make her dream come true at the Chicago marathon.

In addition to running, Rommy works out with weights. "I look better than ever! I have worked hard to define my body through resistance training and am thrilled with the results. I have never felt so toned and athletic!"

To maintain focus, Rommy writes down her weight and exercise program on a calendar every morning and places her progress chart on the refrigerator. "Overall, the key to my success has been planning ahead so that diet and exercise became an easy, convenient part of my life.

"I've inspired my mother to begin the program and hope to show others that becoming your best self is a process that is enjoyable and fulfilling."

Change your life today! Log on to www.biggestloserclub.com and get started.

who started the show at more than 400 pounds," says Neil Tejwani, Season 4. "I see that picture every day. There is a quote underneath it that says, 'Hard? It's supposed to be hard. That's what makes it great.' Losing weight was the hardest thing I've ever done in my life. I don't want to forget about all the aches and pains of being on *The Biggest Loser*; the road I took to get here was not easy. It's not supposed to be easy."

Make Time for Exercise

Most people—and research confirms this—say that a lack of time is the biggest obstacle to their exercising. Truth be told, it's not that we don't have time, it's that we need to use the time we have more effectively. There are 168 hours in a week. Should you be able to squeeze in at least three or four 1-hour workouts? Absolutely!

One way to do it is to "sneak" exercise into your life. Andrea "Drea" Baptiste, Season 1, for example, incorporates exercise into everything she does. "If I'm out and about and I know my next destination is a few blocks away, instead of hailing a cab or driving around the corner, I walk. Instead of checking my bag at the airport and going on the moving walkway, I carry my suitcase, which weighs about 50 pounds."

Pete Thomas believes there are certain

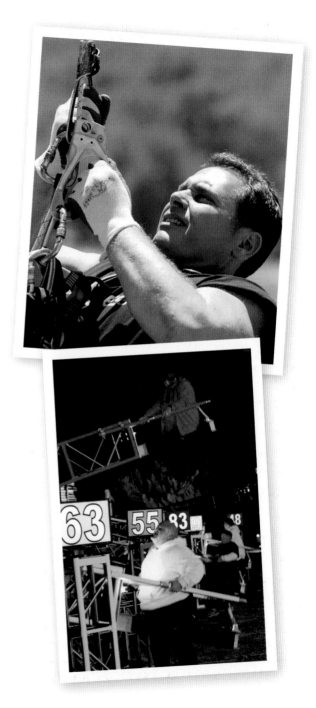

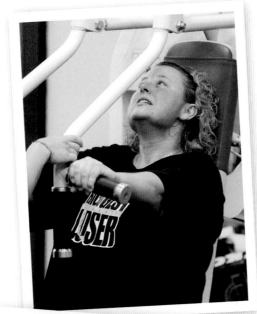

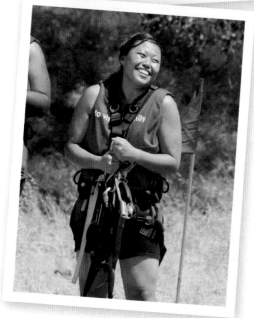

exercises you can do *anywhere*. "I have a group of people I work out with. One of the women in our group takes her child to band practice, which is held at the school where we exercise. She'll drop her child off at practice, then join us at the track for a run. Say your child has a swim meet or some other event at a school. There's no reason why you can't go jogging on the school's track, or find a place to do situps and pushups. You can make time for exercise, or sneak it in, if you commit to finding time for it."

Another way to sneak exercise into your life is to invest in a baby jogger if you're a parent. New parents Suzy Preston and Matt Hoover, Season 2, say this is a great way to exercise as a family. "We put our son, Rex, in a baby jogger and go out for a jog as a family. And by the way, for every hour of holding, feeding, and dressing a baby, you can burn around 200 calories. Being a parent can be good exercise!" Suzy says.

Finding the hours or minutes in the day for a workout is always challenging. One solution is to get up an hour earlier and exercise first thing in the morning. "As life is for most people, I'm very busy," says Jay Kruger, Season 5. "I leave my house at 6:30 a.m. to go to work, and I get home at 5:30 p.m. I've got two little ones who I want to spend time with before they go to bed at 7:30. My solution for fitting in exercise is to do it first thing in the morning. You may have to get up an hour or a half hour earlier than you normally would."

Another benefit to working out in the morning is that you get your workout over with before your day even starts—and that feels good. Plus, exercise energizes you mentally and physically for the rest of the day and boosts your calorie-burning power for the entire day. Circuit training, which is recommended in *The Biggest Loser Fitness Program*, can be performed at a variety of intensity levels, from beginner to expert. Studies have proven that training at higher intensity levels boots your calorie burn for 24 hours or more after your workout. To get in even more exercise, plan times to be physically active with your family, such as a softball game, a weekend hike through a park, or an evening walk around the block.

Another tip if you're time challenged: try to combine movements. For a total-body exercise, incorporate 3- to 5-pound free weights into your cardio training. If you're on the treadmill, for example, pump your arms and shoulders doing overhead presses. That way, you can basically squeeze a cardio and strength-training routine into a 40-minute workout.

Exercising is so vital to shedding pounds, staying fit, and being healthy that you should try to make it a priority. This takes a focused mindset, a steely commitment to doing it—an attitude that Kelly MacFarland has had since she dropped 72 pounds in Season 1. "Exercise is the one thing I won't blow off," she says. "There have been times when I've turned down dates or dinners with my friends because the event would conflict with my workout. At the end of the day when I

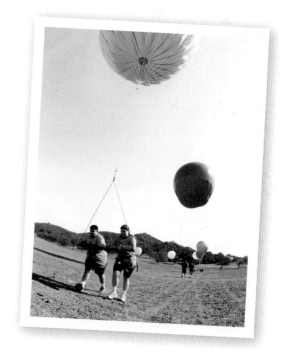

lay my head down, I feel better knowing that I took good care of *me*."

One way to start prioritizing your workout is to write your workout schedule in your day planner or electronic organizer and treat it as you would any other appointment. Don't let other priorities crowd out this important part of your day.

One more time-saving strategy: Have you ever considered exercising while watching TV? It's a tactic employed effectively by Bill Germanakos, the Biggest Loser of Season 4. "Think about it. No matter how busy you get, you still have time for television. Why not combine watching TV with exercising? While watching TV, hop on an exercise bike or any cardio equipment that elevates your heart rate and sustains it so that you burn fat. Or use hand weights or a stability ball while enjoying your favorite TV show."

Mix It Up for Motivation

Repeating the same activity day after day puts you at risk for overuse injuries and could stall your weight loss. Try breaking up one cardio session into a few different workouts—20 minutes of walking, 20 minutes on the bike, 20 minutes climbing stairs or rowing—or doing different types of exercise each time you weight train. Don't get stuck doing the same routine until it becomes stale.

Marty Wolff's exercise routine is a good example. "I really don't have any sort of favorite exercise," says the Season 3 contestant. "I just like moving in general, and I try to do a lot of different activities. My training program now is easy (compared to what I did on the show). I do 4 to 6 hours of cardio a week and lift weights two or three times a week. For cardio, I need a variety because I have attention span problems. I like to run, bike, hike, play sports, and row. Then there's tennis. I enjoy getting competitive and playing tennis with Amy! I usually win!

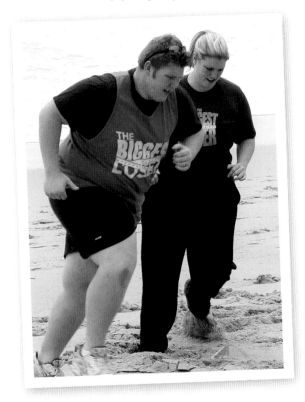

"To the normal person this may seem like a lot of working out, but for a formerly obese person who gains weight fast, it is the best option for me. Working out allows me to not be a prisoner to my diet. I'm able to be more lenient on certain days, and let's face it, if I want ice cream a couple days a week, I eat ice cream. I still keep track of calories, but I can be more indulgent if I've done my workout. I now have the tools to manage my healthy lifestyle, and exercise is one of them."

As Marty points out, the key is to do different activities. For example, you might want to try a sport instead of conventional exercise, periodically change the sequence and types of exercises in your routine, try different classes, or participate in fitness challenges sponsored by your gym or health club.

Possibly one of the most unusual and varied routines is employed by Season 4 *Biggest Loser* cast member David Griffin. "What works best for me is functional exercise that mimics how the body performs daily activities," he says. "My trainer and I beat tractor tires with sledgehammers, for example. We flip tractor tires, carry them, and drag them. We run around with sandbags. We run bleachers. These activities make for a really hard, but fun workout. There are a lot of things you can do besides traditional exercises like weight lifting or using cardio equipment."

But what happens if you start feeling bored with your exercise choices? Isabeau Miller, Season 4 finalist, suggests trying something competitive. "Train for, and compete in, a race. This will break up the monotony. I ran my first 5-K last year, and

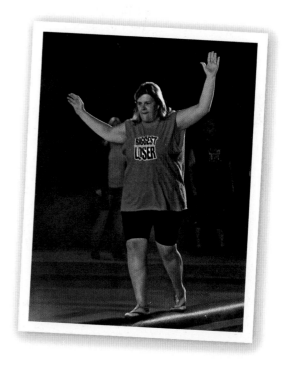

now I'm planning on training for a 10-K and potentially a half-marathon. In addition to alleviating exercise boredom, there is nothing like the adrenaline rush you feel crossing the finish line and having people cheer for you."

Another strategy to prevent the exercise doldrums from setting in is to explore new exercise techniques. Take the recent trend toward kettle bell workouts, for example. These cast-iron weights, which resemble cannonballs, are a form of weight training that was popular at the turn of the previous century and is now making a comeback. "I love them!" says Kelly MacFarland, Season 1. "Using kettle bells, you can build core strength, burn fat, sculpt your body, and create an overall athletic physique."

Kelly also likes to check out different gyms to stave off exercise boredom. "I've become a gym rat anyway, so I'm comfortable in any gym. This helps get me out of my comfort zone and provides new challenges."

No matter what activity or activities you choose, Season 4's Biggest Loser Bill Germanakos advises that you use a calorie-burn counter to keep you motivated. "You wear the device on your arm," he explains. "Basically, it calculates your calorie burn throughout the day by measuring stuff like the number of steps you take and your body temperature. Before bed, you can upload the information to your computer, log what you ate that day, and learn what your calorie deficit (or surplus) is. If you want to lose, say, a pound a week, you have to burn 500 calories more than you consume daily. It's a great way to monitor how many calories you've burned through exercise, and it motivates you to burn more."

BIGGEST LOSER TOOLBOX

"When it comes to losing weight, you will take out of it whatever you choose to put into it. If you work out half an hour a day, a few days a week, you can't expect the same results you'd get from 1 hour a day, 6 days a week. If you put in half-hearted work, you'll get half-hearted results."

—Isabeau Miller, Season 4 finalist

Exercise: Getting Started

We hope these strategies help you get in gear. In the words of *Biggest Loser* twins Bill and Jim Germanakos from Season 4, "If you want to get it done, you've got to get it started." How true! For many people, though, the toughest part about starting an exercise routine is just that: starting. If the idea of doing 60 minutes of solid exercise feels too overwhelming, try starting with 10-minute segments at a time and then gradually build up from there. Once you combine two chunks of 10 minutes, you're doing 20 minutes, and then you can add another 10 to make it 30, and you're on your way. While it's true that most guidelines recommend doing 30 to 60 minutes of exercise on most days of the week, this amount might be unrealistic for you initially. So take small steps every day, be faithful about it, and soon you'll be hooked on an active lifestyle.

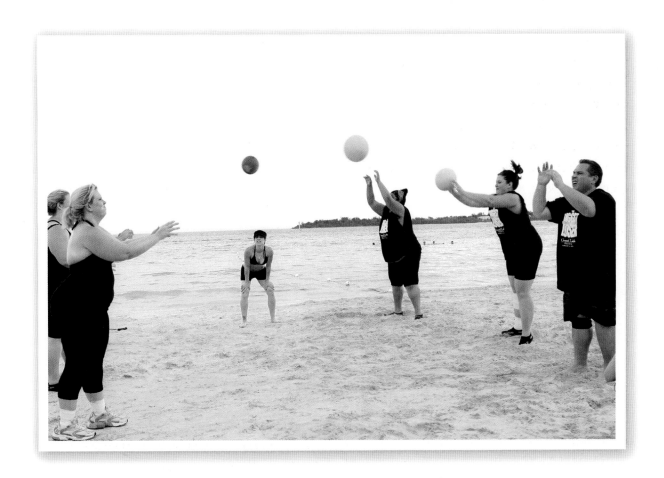

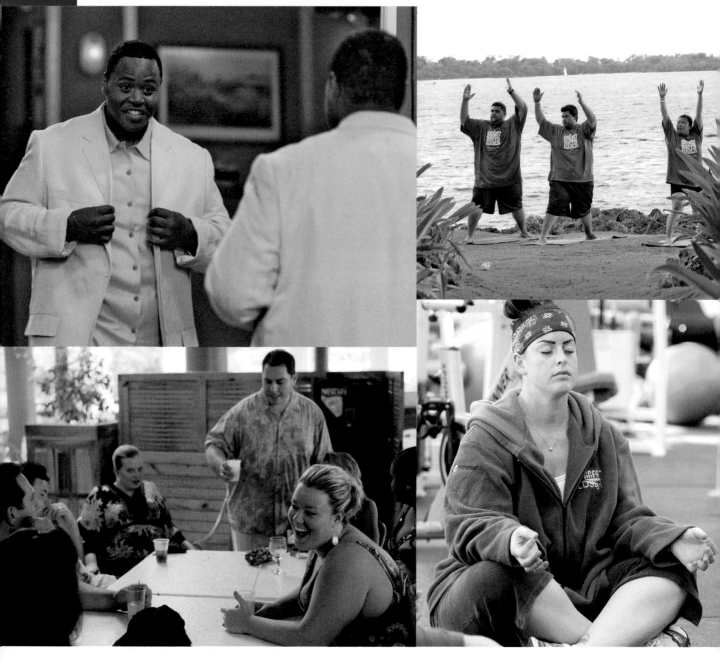

Managing Self-Esteem and Body Image Issues: Tips for Staying Positive and Strong

When you think about it, the process of losing weight focuses mostly on numbers: calories eaten and burned, hours exercised, pounds lost. But numbers don't tell the whole story. The way you feel about yourself and your appearance also plays an important part in reaching your goals.

But therein lies a problem. We live in a world focused on body image—the perfect body image, that is. Women are constantly reminded to be slender but curvaceous; men are supposed to be muscular, yet lean. But most of us are just ordinary mortals with our fair share of cellulite, tummy rolls, and other "flaws." Surveys indicate that about one-third of us don't like how we

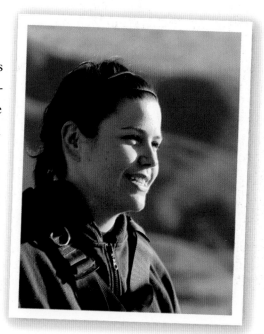

look, women more so than men. Women are most unhappy with their thighs, bellies, breasts, and buttocks. Men tend to be dissatisfied with their abdomens or pectorals. Sometimes the desire to lose weight has more to do with wanting these specific body parts to be "perfect" than with the desire to be fit and healthy. More likely than not, you have at least one body part that bugs you, and it's easy to get frustrated when it doesn't look the way you want it to, despite your diligent diet and exercise routine.

But bashing your body takes a toll on the rest of you, too. When you feel miserable about yourself, you're less inclined to take care of your body by nourishing it with healthy foods or going to the gym. Poor body image—the negative views you hold about your body's size and proportions—also leads to unrealistic and sometimes unhealthy weight-loss goals. Instead of focusing on having a perfectly flat stomach, for instance, your goal should be to build your core strength. A flatter stomach will come in time, but it shouldn't be the goal. Your body needs time to process all of the changes you are making, and it may take a while before you start to see the results of your hard work—especially if you have a significant amount of weight to lose. Setting goals based on perceived body flaws will only lead to disappointment and kill your motivation down the road. You don't want or need that. Cultivating a healthier attitude about your body paves the way for success, and your confidence will extend into your weight-loss efforts. Every season, *The Biggest Loser* cast members—some of whom lose more than 100 pounds—learn to love their bodies, flaws and all—and so can you.

You Are Unique: Don't Compare Yourself

The appearance-obsessed world we live in makes it tough to love our bodies. It's important to remember that there's no such thing as an "ideal" body, and that different cultures have different standards and norms for appropriate body size and shape. Even within a particular culture, societal standards shift periodically. In certain South Pacific island cultures, for example, a person's extra weight is considered a sign of affluence and elevated social status, but that same person would be termed obese in the United States, where a slim

> ### BIGGEST LOSER TOOLBOX
>
> "If you gain back some weight, don't beat yourself up over it. Instead, focus on how much you've lost and how far you've come. Then get back on track."
> —Andrea Overstreet, Season 2

and trim physique is worshipped. Trying to live up to these standards can be very damaging, because few of us can attain a "perfect" body, no matter how it is defined.

Kae Whang, Season 4, has dealt with this pressure throughout her entire life. "As an Asian

BIGGEST LOSER TOOLBOX

"Look in the mirror every day and be proud of where you are."
　　　　　　—Isabeau Miller, Season 4 finalist

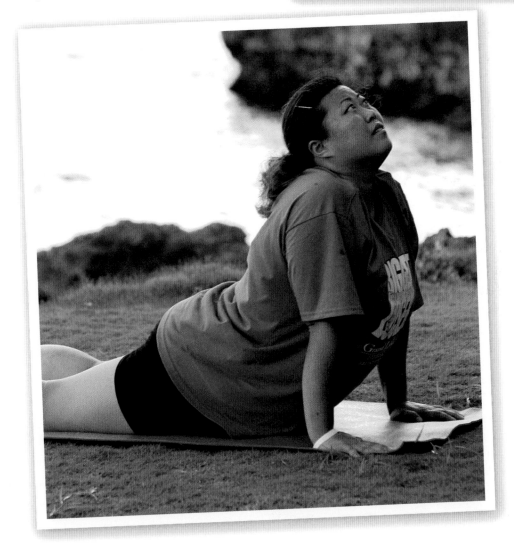

female, I've felt pressured to conform to the Asian stereotype of being very thin. Because I never was, I didn't feel like a complete person. At the same time, I was stereotyped because I was overweight. I was so overwhelmed that I stopped caring about my looks, and I wore frumpy clothes. I used to be so nervous just going out in public because I thought people were judging me all the time. But now, I've worked so hard that I don't care what other people think. That's a great attitude to adopt."

Comparing your body to someone else's can get in the way of progress. If you're too caught up in what everybody else looks like or is able to do, then you'll forget what you're doing and accomplishing, and that's what really matters. "I was in

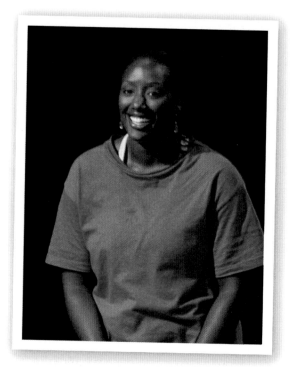

Best Moment: Ali Vincent, Season 5

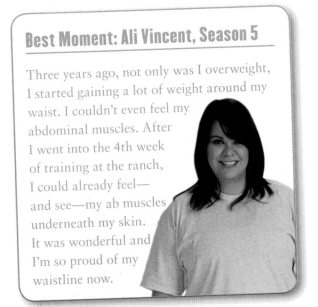

Three years ago, not only was I overweight, I started gaining a lot of weight around my waist. I couldn't even feel my abdominal muscles. After I went into the 4th week of training at the ranch, I could already feel—and see—my ab muscles underneath my skin. It was wonderful and I'm so proud of my waistline now.

Las Vegas recently, sunning myself out by the pool, wearing my bikini, and thinking I'm the hottest thing out there," recalls Season 1's Andrea "Drea" Baptiste. "Then a woman with a Barbie-like figure strolls by, and I'm thinking *Arrgghh.* All of a sudden I noticed a little spread in my hips, a wrinkle here and there, and some cellulite—until I snapped myself back into common sense. Regardless of what imperfections are there, I love me for who I am. My body and I are pals. That's how I look at it. Gaining self-acceptance doesn't mean changing your body as much as it means changing your mind-set."

Make Peace with Your Body

The process of making peace with your body is a skill, and like any other skill, it has to be learned and then practiced, practiced, practiced. As with any new habit, it gets easier and more intuitive with experience. When you're truly at peace with yourself, you'll find that you're less prone to give in to emotional eating and you'll feel genuinely connected to yourself and your healthy lifestyle.

A surefire way to start making peace with your body is with a little self-nurturing. Aim to give yourself at least 20 to 30 minutes of private time every day to do something that makes you feel better in mind and body. It could be as simple as soaking in the tub after a grueling workout, putting lotion on your newly toned legs, or finding a quiet place to meditate or listen to your favorite music. Private time is one of the best ways to help you treat yourself, which you deserve whether you feel you've "earned" it or not, and feeling good will boost your chances of sticking to your program.

"I learned to start taking care of my appearance with makeup, a new hairstyle, and skin cream, even when I had lots of pounds to lose," says Kae Whang, Season 4. "Your physical appearance makes a statement about who you are and how you feel about yourself. If you look slovenly, you will feel slovenly. If you look terrible in your clothes, you feel terrible. If you don't feel good about the way you look, it is difficult to feel confident, energetic, or motivated. The more attractive you can make yourself look, the more confidence you will exude."

Another tool that can help improve your body image is exercise. Being a couch potato breeds self-criticism. As soon as you get active, no matter what your size, you'll begin feeling better about yourself, and eventually you'll see results that will help you appreciate your body even more. Says Bernie Salazar, Season 5, "There were times in my life during which I just felt beat up and discouraged

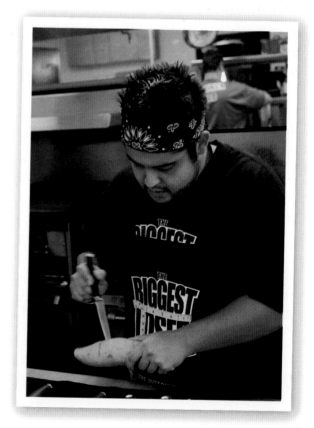

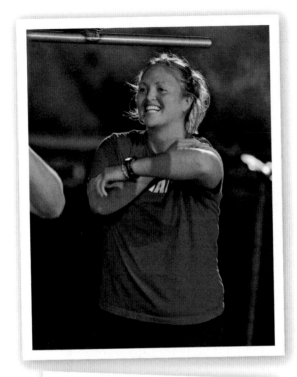

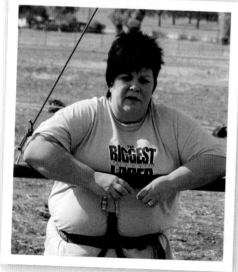

by my weight. Instead of doing something about it, I'd eat more, seclude myself more, and just sit around feeling moody—can you relate? But once I started exercising, I felt a real sense of accomplishment."

Keep in mind, too, that so much of what you look like—your basic body shape and composition—is under genetic control. "You can remodel the 'house' you were born with to some extent, but you can't rebuild the foundation," says Pam Smith, Season 3. "Accept what you've inherited, appreciate it, and know that you're making the best of who you are and what you look like."

It's important to accept where you are today. If you appreciate each point in your journey, you'll harness the positive energy it takes to achieve your goal weight. Says Bette-Sue Burklund, Season 5, "I used to fall in the trap of thinking, 'I'll be happy when I lose 50 or 75 pounds.' That way of thinking made it hard for me to achieve my goal and

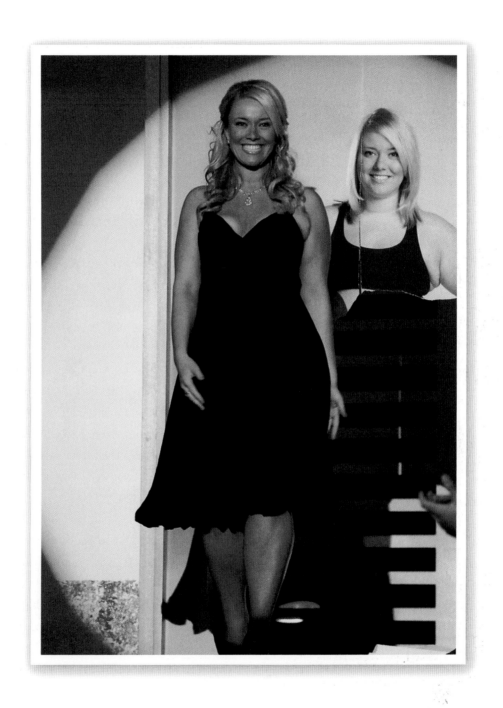

If you believe that you can't be happy or satisfied until you are thin, you will be more likely to give up out of present-moment dissatisfaction and frustration with yourself. But if you can say, "I eventually want to be thinner, but in the meantime I can be happy with myself and enjoy my body and my looks the way they are now," you're much more likely to sail past any bumps in the road between where you are today and your goal. On *The Biggest Loser* you've seen overweight, out-of-shape people rise to all kinds of amazing physical challenges and, in the process, come to value and appreciate their bodies in ways they never could

stay there. Why? Because I delayed happiness and self-satisfaction—a negative state of mind that made me feel like a failure—with no real push to help me get to that goal."

The Biggest Loser Online Club Profile: **Sara Crank**

Starting weight: 260 • Current weight: 189.9 • Goal weight: 150

"After eating my way through my divorce and ballooning to 260 pounds, I knew I needed a change, but I just didn't have the motivation to do it," says Sara, age 26.

She got help from her best friend, Jim, who told her that if she really wanted to shed 100 pounds, he would move to her town to help her.

"I started this journey for that reason, but after altering my diet and changing my eating habits, I realized that this journey is for me and to improve my life and the life of my son."

Exercising helped her take off nearly 70 pounds, and she ran her first 5-K race on Memorial Day. "It was an amazing experience," she says. "I ran it in 37:34, which is 4 minutes quicker than my personal best. I now run an average of 5 miles a day and I feel amazing. This has just been an awesome, life-changing journey, and I love it!"

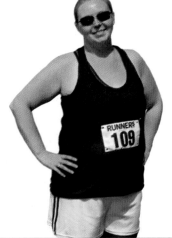

Change your life today! Log on to www.biggestloserclub.com and get started.

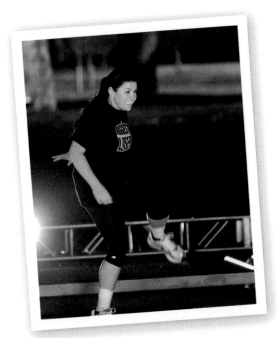

proud of my strength and endurance. I can outrun most people who weigh less than I do. I can take my personal trainer boyfriend through a workout that even he can't survive. I can train for 2 hours and not get tired! Yes, I do feel that I look so much different, but most importantly I feel very strong, and I'm ready to accomplish anything."

The mirror can be your best friend or your worst enemy when you're trying to make peace with your body. It depends on how you "talk back" to your reflection. "The next time you look in the mirror, say something nice, even if you have to

have imagined. Try to love all the good things your body does for *you*, whether that's winning a game of miniature golf, playing with your kids, or salsa dancing with your partner. How could you enjoy physical activity and movement without your body?

Isabeau Miller, Season 4 finalist, agrees: "I'm proud of not just what my body looks like, but what it can do. At first I didn't recognize how much I had changed. Last year, I visited my mom in New York City. After a few hours of walking around, I was totally exhausted. When I visited her this year, we did the same thing again, but I felt just fine. It's little things like that that can go unappreciated and you often take for granted. I'm

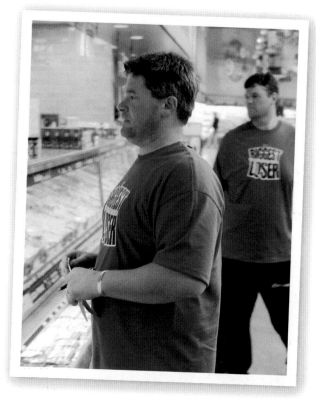

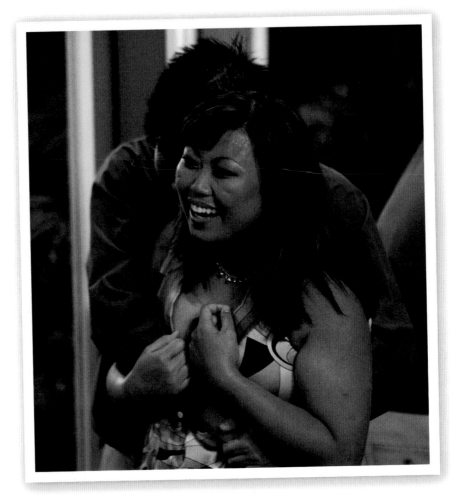

force it at first," advises Brittany Aberle, Season 5. Try "My waist is beautiful," "My hips are just right," or her personal favorite, "I'm steamy hot!"

Kae Whang, Season 4, feels the same way. "Sometimes I forget that I've lost weight, and that 225-pound girl reappears in my mind. But then I look in the mirror, and I see that I did lose that weight. You do get those old feelings and insecuri-ties again, but you have to stop and say, 'No.' Remember what you went through and that you are now strong and confident. It is amazing how much your mentality will change afterward."

Your reflection in the mirror can also be a reality check. Mark Kruger, Season 5, explains, "My brother Jay and I were at a ball game at Fen-way Park when the casting director for *The Big-*

gest Loser approached us and asked if we wanted to be on the show. I knew I was heavy, but I didn't know I was heavy enough to get on *The Biggest Loser*! That night I looked in the mirror—it was a reality check—and admitted to myself that I should do something about my weight before it got worse. Now I never want to go back to where I was. When I look in the mirror now, I feel a lot better about what I see looking back at me."

Set Reasonable Goals

When you begin a weight-loss program, you usually have a specific goal weight you want to reach. You may also be hoping to achieve a physique like those of the trim, toned celebrities you see in the media. But the photos of the bodies that smile out at you from the pages of the glossies are airbrushed and modified with software to make them look

> ### Toughest Moment:
> ### Trent Patterson, Season 5
>
> Five months before I went to the ranch, my wife and I had a baby, so it was rough for me to be away from home. I just kept telling myself that I was losing weight and getting healthy for them, and that helped me make the best of each day at the ranch.

flawless. Instead of being distracted by them, focus on *your* body and how you can make it the best it can be—then go about achieving your goal in a healthful way.

Says Kae Whang, Season 4, "I think it's terrible that women think they have to starve to look a certain way—you know, like the models in the fashion magazines. I've learned that you don't have to starve to get thinner. You can actually eat five times a day and the weight will come off if you exercise. Fortunately, there's a new trend in the media in which stronger, athletic women are being featured more prominently, and I love that. That's what a real woman should look like. Personally, I know I am healthy now. I don't need to be a skinny,

> ### BIGGEST LOSER TOOLBOX
>
> "Sometimes when I get in a slump or feel frustrated about my weight or think 'Oh, it's just easier to be fat,' I stop the thought with 'No, I want to conquer this negativity now.'"
>
> —Suzy Preston, Season 2 finalist

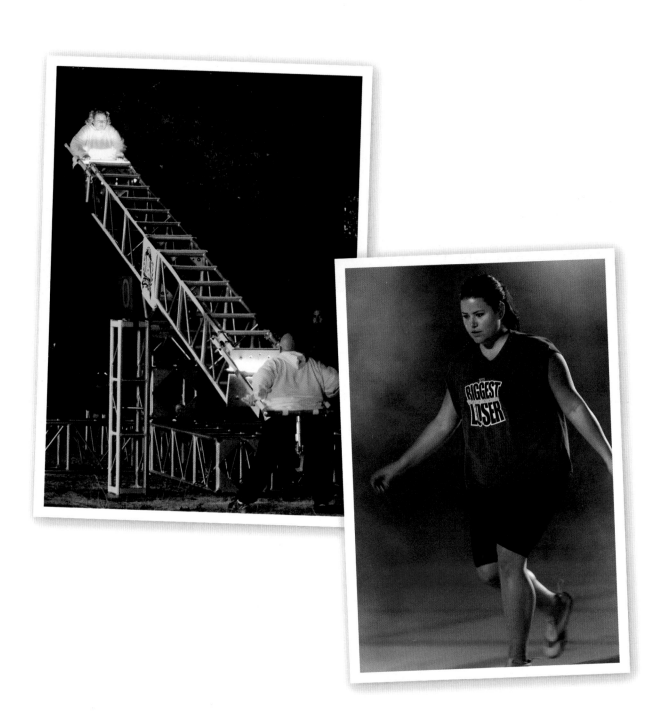

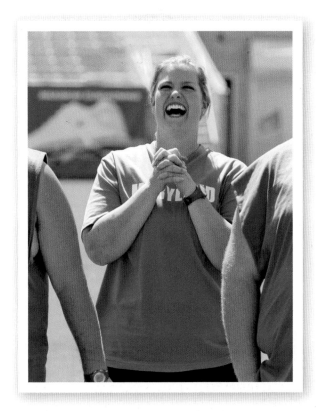

statement with something more positive and rational, such as "Every moment I exercise and eat right, my body is becoming stronger and more efficient." This kind of self-talk will help you to banish destructive habits.

As you're losing weight, give yourself credit for all the little milestones you reach along the way, especially in your workouts. This could be an extra mile walked, a drop in blood pressure, or a better night's sleep. "I've been amazed at what I've accomplished," says Julie Hadden, Season 4 runner-up. "I can't believe a body can physically go through so much and survive. For most of us on *The Biggest Loser*, it is the first time we have felt proud of ourselves in a long time. No amount of money can measure up to having self-esteem. Not even $250,000."

Before being a finalist on *The Biggest Loser* in Season 4, Isabeau Miller didn't have much hope for her career, although her dream was to be a singer-songwriter. Instead of going to Nashville

bony, fragile size 0. I appreciate myself now because I'm strong and healthy, and I lead a fulfilling life."

Stay Inwardly Positive

Your innermost conversations can have a powerful impact on your body image and motivation. What you think determines what you say, what you do, and how you act. Constantly telling yourself "I'm too fat" is a defeatist attitude. Replace that type of

BIGGEST LOSER TOOLBOX

"When I lapse into negative thinking, I go out and drown myself in positive friends who make me laugh. Laughter is definitely a cure-all."

—Andrea "Drea" Baptiste, Season 1

and meeting people, she sat on the couch and told herself, "Oh, maybe I'll be a real estate agent." She says, "I was afraid to go for anything because I was afraid of failing. I told myself I couldn't make it."

Isabeau changed her self-talk as she changed her weight. "I'm starting to perform in Nashville, which I never would have had the courage to do before, and I've met with a big music executive already."

Kelly Fields, Season 5, believes it is important to start "thinking thin." As she started to lose weight, she began to think of herself as thin and see herself as slimmer, active, and pretty. "This has helped me adjust my attitude to a new, more positive image of myself. My old fat self may want more to eat, but my new thin self knows it does not need more. This new, improved image of myself has helped supply the necessary motivation to keep going."

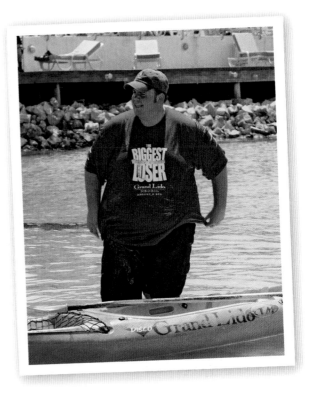

As Brittany Aberle began her Season 5 journey on *The Biggest Loser*, she moved deep into a healthful lifestyle, eating much better than ever and pushing her body with intense bouts of exercise. "The pounds started to melt off and my ability to love myself blossomed. When I looked in the mirror, I actually liked what I saw. Now I feel strong, empowered, and proud of myself for taking control of my life—not just my weight. It's interesting because this increase in self-esteem, in turn, helped me keep up my new exercise and eating habits, which then helped me feel more confi-

> ### BIGGEST LOSER TOOLBOX
>
> "Believe you can be someone different than what you see in the mirror. Meditate and visualize about how wonderful the future can be. You owe it to yourself and to everybody who loves you."
>
> —Julie Hadden, Season 4 runner-up

dent. And though I have times when I still think my belly is too big, most of the time I view my body with pride."

More Words of *Biggest Loser* Wisdom

Sure, there are going to be times when you want to throw in the towel. When that happens, try a technique that has worked for Amy Hildreth, Season 3: Write yourself a love letter. "To keep myself motivated, I wrote down how my life would improve and change if I became more active and lost weight. During hard times, I would take it out, read it, and encourage myself," she says.

Remarkably, Isabeau Miller, Season 4 finalist, has managed to maintain a no-quitting mentality through all the ups and downs of getting in shape. "Quitting? That option was gone the minute I donned spandex on national TV. I told myself, 'I *will* make it through the impossible. I *will* come out stronger and wiser, happier, and healthier. I will *not ever* forget the way I was. I will not let myself lose faith that God put me here for a reason. I have a purpose to fulfill and hopefully, someday, I'll know what that purpose is.'"

Enjoy the compliments you receive, too—and you *will* be receiving them. Your first impulse may be to modestly downplay any praise, but when

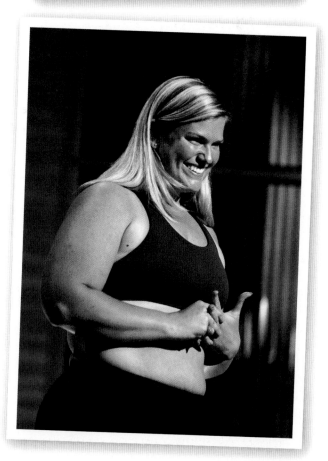

someone compliments you, accept it graciously and know that you deserve those words. Says Season 4's David Griffin, "It sure feels nice when people comment, 'Wow, you look like a different person.' I see people I've known for years and they give me second and third looks. They see a guy who's generally healthy. It does give me a feeling of pride and accomplishment that I'm being recognized for the fruits of my labor. Of course, I still see a lot of work to be done. But even if you can't yet see your success with your own eyes, you can see it through other people's eyes. It still feels great."

Finally, keep in mind that you have intelligence, feelings, and spirit. You are more than just your body—you are a multidimensional human being taking control of your own destiny—and *that* is something worth celebrating.

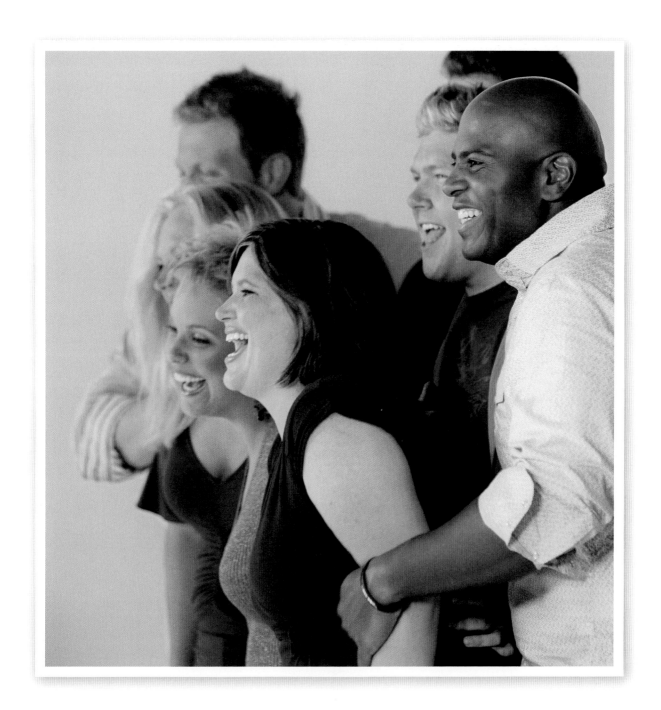

5

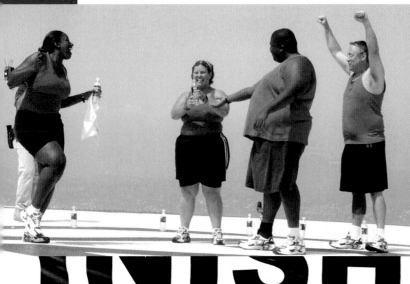
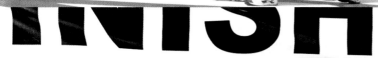
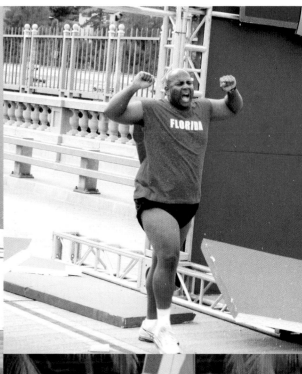
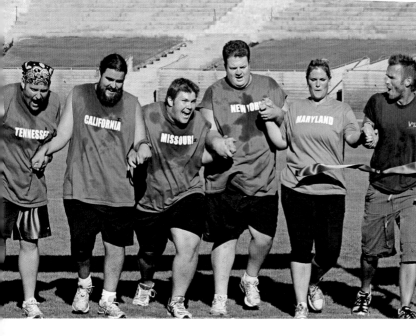
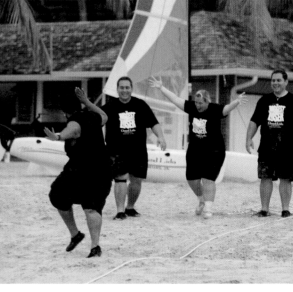

Staying in the Game: Inspiration to Help You Reach Your Goals

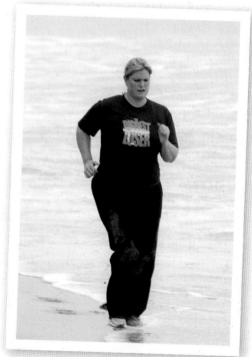

How often have you said to yourself, "I can't stick to my diet" or "I'll skip my workout today," and the next thing you know, several days have passed without so much as a situp or a salad? Getting in shape takes too much work and too much time to see results. Or does it?

We've all been there—even the cast members of *The Biggest Loser*. No matter how hard you try to stick with your get-in-shape plan, you find yourself dreaming of chocolate cake instead of vegetables or lounging in front of the TV instead of hoofing it on the treadmill. Pretty soon your plan bites the dust and you slip back into your old habits.

So—where can you get the staying power to see your plan through this time? Some of the best advice you'll find on staying motivated is right here, straight from the cast members who have struggled with—and conquered—this very issue, and kept off hundreds of pounds as a result. Rescue yourself from motivational quicksand with their stick-to-it strategies.

Put Your Goals on Paper

Seeing is believing and achieving—so write down your goals and keep a visible reminder of them in front of you. Place your list of goals on your bathroom mirror, on your refrigerator door, by your computer, at your desk, in your car, or wherever you spend a lot of time. "This helps you visualize where you want to go and sets your mind on getting there," says Amy Hildreth, Season 3.

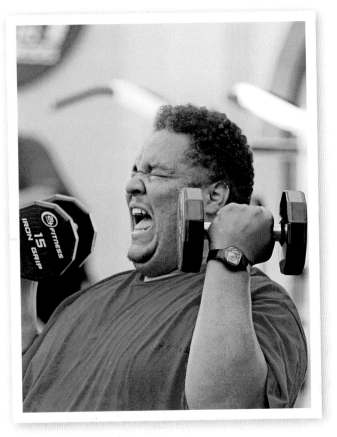

BIGGEST LOSER TOOLBOX

"Eating too fast causes you to eat more. I've learned to eat more slowly and drink water with my meals, so that the feeling of satisfaction will register better."
—Jenn Widder, Season 5

Pete Thomas, Season 2, believes in writing down two sets of goals: one for losing weight and the other for keeping it off. "As soon as you've lost the weight, begin to work on the second set," he says. "To keep the weight off, you're going to apply some of the same principles from the first set. Your calorie intake, for example, may have gone up by 500 calories a day, but you've still got to eat quality food, not skip meals, drink plenty of water, and work out most days of the week."

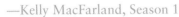
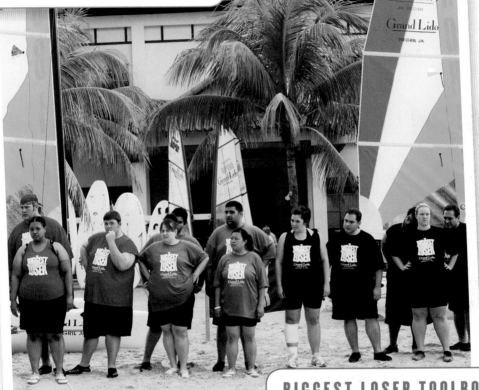

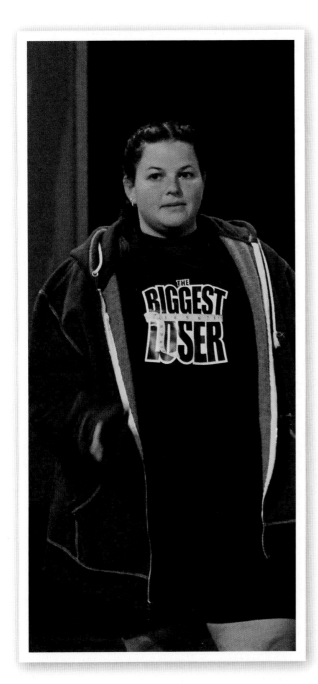

"Most of my negative thoughts rear their ugly heads when the numbers on the scale are low after I've worked really hard. I start feeling like everything I'm doing isn't good enough. But I've learned to be proud of any loss I have, and I pat myself on the back for it. Then I remember all the weight I've already lost. That's a good feeling."
—Jenn Widder, Season 5

When writing down your goals, make sure they're SMART:

Specific

Measurable

Action-based

Realistic and Rewarding

Time-based

"*Specific* and *measurable* mean that you can evaluate whether or not you have reached the goal by answering yes or no," explains *The Biggest Loser* Online Club expert Greg Hottinger. "*Action-based* means that you can see yourself doing it. *Realistic* means you have the skills, knowledge, and tools to make it happen. *Rewarding* means you find it exciting and valuable. And *time-based* makes it closed-ended, so you can't continually delay the start or move the finish line."

Put In the Work—You're Worth It

Most people start any new task with over-the-top enthusiasm. At first, everything is exciting. But underneath those good intentions, doubt creeps in from every angle. Marty Wolff, Season 3, knows this feeling all too well. "I was at a place in my life where I didn't feel worthy of change," he says. "What *The Biggest Loser* ultimately taught me is that I am worth losing the weight and that I can do anything I put my mind and my heart to."

Marty has a simple suggestion for staying

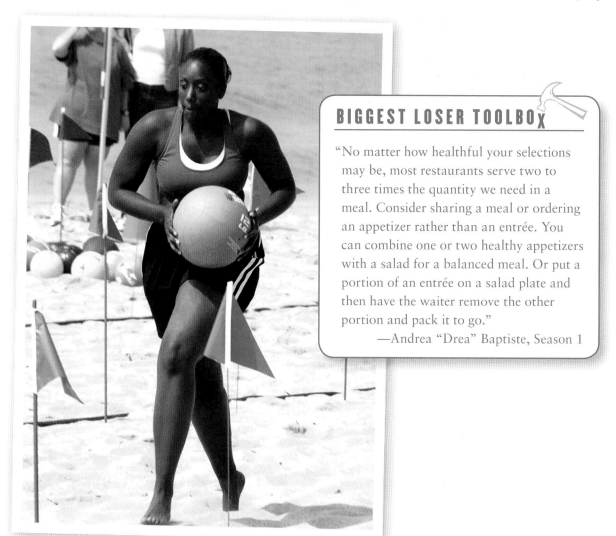

BIGGEST LOSER TOOLBOX

"No matter how healthful your selections may be, most restaurants serve two to three times the quantity we need in a meal. Consider sharing a meal or ordering an appetizer rather than an entrée. You can combine one or two healthy appetizers with a salad for a balanced meal. Or put a portion of an entrée on a salad plate and then have the waiter remove the other portion and pack it to go."

—Andrea "Drea" Baptiste, Season 1

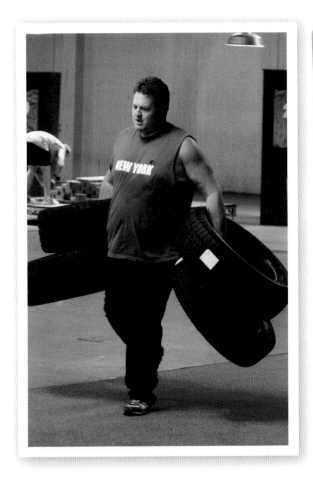

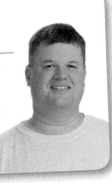
Take Small, Manageable Steps

For some of us, the most effective way to adopt new eating and exercise habits is by taking small, conservative steps—no abrupt changes in lifestyle or behavior. No grandiose pledges to lose 20 pounds in a month, or to exercise super-hard for hours every day, or to never eat cheesecake again. Small steps, successfully completed, build confidence. Or as Trent Patterson, Season 5, puts it, "Take it one day at a time, and make the best out of each day."

Isabeau Miller, Season 4 finalist, suggests making little changes every day for a month. "Too many weight-loss programs want you to make huge, wholesale changes overnight. That can be overwhelming. Just make one or two changes at a time, like eating fresh fruit or vegetables, cutting out processed foods, or starting a walking program. After a month, step back, look at your progress, and appreciate what you've achieved."

motivated so you won't slip back into old habits: Constantly ask yourself, What kind of life do I want to live? "Once you answer that question, you can create an action plan, with SMART goals, to get there," he says. "Keep revisiting that plan. It gives you a clear direction of where you need to go, and you'll stay motivated. Make sure you do something every day to get there."

Use Your Tools to Break Old Habits

Why are bad habits so hard to break? Over time, our unhealthy tendencies (such as overeating or smoking) become habitual, learned behaviors. In other words, we fall back into them practically without thinking. One of the keys to overcoming these weaknesses is to replace them with new, healthful intentions day after day after day, so that those new behaviors become routine. Use the "Biggest Loser Toolbox" eating and exercise tips highlighted throughout this chapter to make this process happen. "External discipline—using your tools—creates internal discipline, which leads to the formation of better habits," says Season 2's Pete Thomas.

Learn the Power of *No*

If you're like most people, you say yes to too many requests and demands. Saying yes to everything that is asked of you creates pressure—and pressure-related overeating. Suzy Preston, Season 2 finalist, is one cast member who knows a lot about saying yes too much and no not enough. She realized that when she got home from the ranch, she was going to have a tougher time protecting her workouts and her eating preferences and limiting her availability to others. It's still a balancing act for her.

"At the ranch, there was no one for me to please," she says. "I swung in the other direction and got really selfish. It was all about me. Then I got home and I was like a fish out of water. I couldn't go back to the way I was before *The Biggest Loser*, but I couldn't be the way I was at the ranch."

A new Suzy definitely emerged, one who takes care of herself and works hard to make sure she never goes back to her old role of only taking care of others. "It's something I deal with all the time. I have a hard time not being all things to all people. My mom helps me realize when I'm falling back into old patterns. Every day I have to check

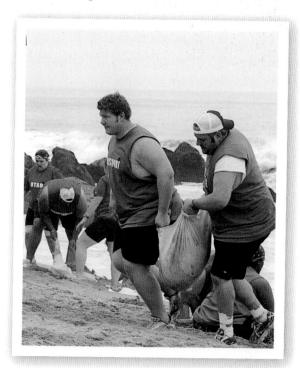

myself. I'm learning to say 'Let me get back to you'
to other people's requests and checking in with
myself—and Matt [Hoover, Season 2]—before I
commit to something new," she says.

Pete Thomas, Season 2, agrees that *no* may be
one of the most powerful words in your weight-
loss vocabulary. "You've got to make up your mind
that *you* are a priority and plan your life accord-
ingly. That means making your health paramount
and learning to say no more often."

Banish Negative Thoughts

In the nooks and crannies of your mind, you have
old "tapes" that tend to be played over and over
again, until finally they represent your version of
the truth. The trouble is, these tapes probably were
recorded so long ago that they may have little to
do with your present situation or direction. And
unfortunately, many of these tapes are negative
and self-destructive. They include criticisms, fears,

irrational thoughts, and put-downs. "If you call
yourself or a part of your body ugly, fat, or dis-
gusting, it registers in your mind just like it would
if someone else said it," says Michael Scholtz, *The
Biggest Loser* Online Club expert.

When one of these negative tapes begins to
play, you may find yourself foraging in the refrigerator for binge food or grabbing some high-calorie
junk food at the drive-through.

Scholtz says that you can turn your inner
voice into an ally to build self-confidence and
a pathway to successful lifestyle change. How?
"If you begin to replace each negative comment
you 'hear' with a positive one, your inner dialogue
will soon be a wall against negative outside
influence and a source of inner peace and resolve,"
he says.

Some examples: Replace "I've tried and I always
fail" with "I don't always fail. Every healthful

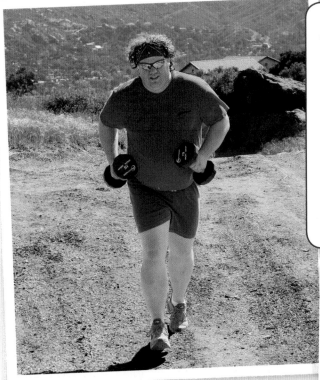

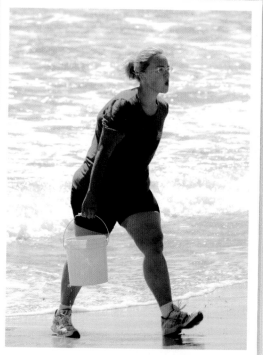

choice I make is a major success." Or replace "I'm not very athletic" with "Regular exercise makes me feel like an athlete." And when doubt creeps in, remind yourself that you have the tools and skills to handle challenges more effectively than you did in the past.

A tape that continued to play in Amy Hildreth's mind during Season 3 was that losing 100 pounds was not even doable. "What seemed

The Biggest Loser Online Club Profile: Michelle Rose

Starting weight: 198 • Current weight: 146 • Goal weight: 120

After joining *The Biggest Loser* Online Club, Michelle realized that the focus is to get healthy. "Losing the weight becomes secondary when you realize how much better you feel by putting smart choices in your mouth," she says. "My cholesterol has dropped over 100 points and my blood pressure is staying in the healthy range now. When people ask me what diet I am on, I tell them I am on *The Biggest Loser* plan, and that it isn't a diet at all, but a common sense approach about making healthy choices."

There are other benefits, too. Michelle says, "I am proud and happy to walk into a store and try things on again. I actually had a bathing suit on last week and went to the pool—something I haven't done in years!"

Michelle's biggest challenge has been cooking. "I did a lot of fast food, boxed meals, and processed foods (all the easy stuff) before starting *The Biggest Loser*. In the beginning, it was really tough, but I realized all I had to do was make double of whatever I was cooking and freeze it. Now I still have boxed meals, but they are healthy and sitting in my freezer just waiting to be heated up when I'm too busy to cook."

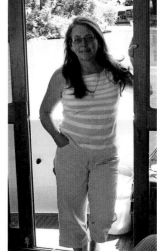

Michelle works out with a close friend who "keeps me motivated when it comes to exercising and just moving in general. It is a lot easier to do with her by my side!"

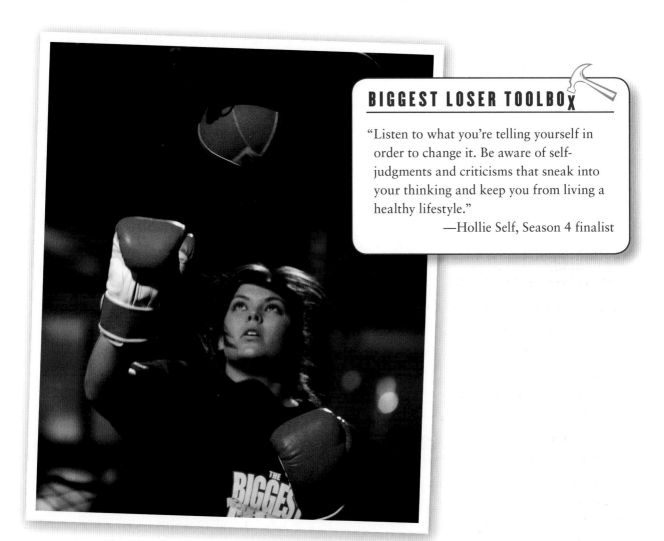

impossible when I looked at it in total—taking off 100 pounds—became manageable when I took it step by step. I learned from my own experience, using the tools and skills, that it is possible to achieve your goal." With that old tape "erased" from her mind, Amy went on to lose 80 pounds.

Other *Biggest Loser* strategies for banishing negative thoughts are featured in the toolboxes throughout this chapter.

Handle Crises

Life is not without crisis—whether it is a divorce, the death of a loved one, a job loss, bankruptcy, or even a minor crisis like bouncing a check or messing up at work. When a crisis hits, as it inevitably will, it is easy to throw your healthy lifestyle out the window and resort to unhealthy behaviors to cope with it. However, the most effective tool for coping with a crisis is to stick to your plan. When you're healthy and energized, you're in better shape to work through and resolve a crisis. Managing a crisis means not letting your healthy choices slide and not letting the crisis immobilize you. "Healthful eating and exercise are really what helps you make it through those times of pain," says Amy Hildreth, Season 3.

What Pete Thomas, Season 2, advises is to have a plan in place to deal with the crises that will erupt in life. "This plan might involve recruiting an accountability person to make sure you get to the gym, even if it is just to talk. When you're in

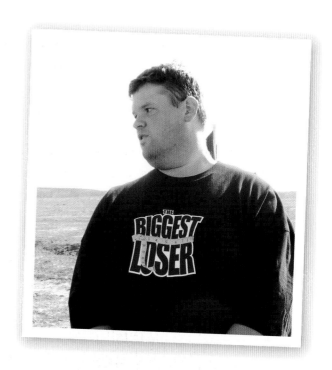

trouble, don't be too proud to ask for help. Or it might involve using stress management techniques to help keep your mind and mood clear. It's really important to keep putting one foot in front of the other—in other words, sticking to your routine. The crisis will pass. You don't want to come out the other side of the crisis having gained 30 pounds. Then you've got another crisis on your hands. If you were able to keep your weight off in the midst of a crisis, that by itself will give you strength to go on."

As Pete notes, it's important to have some stress management strategies to fall back on. You might start employing various relaxation techniques, for example. One of these is massage, which slows the heart rate, relaxes muscles, and relieves pain associated with chronic tension. Other activities that promote relaxation include exercising, listening to soothing music, meditating, practicing breathing techniques, performing progressive muscle relaxation, and doing visualization. Exercises that incorporate both mind and body, such as Pilates, tai chi, and yoga, are also excellent stress relievers. All forms of exercise release endorphins—your body's natural feel-good chemicals—which will help you combat your feelings of anxiety and depression and give you a mental lift.

Stay consistent, too. Your mind will come up with any number of excuses for not exercising or eating healthfully in the midst of a crisis. Don't let these passing thoughts distract you from your

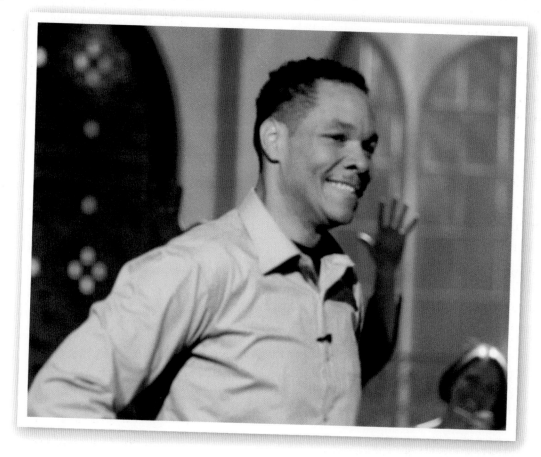

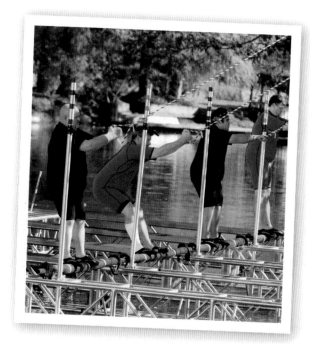

ging a spoon into a gallon container of ice cream during a crisis. But when you eat well, get some physical activity, and practice self-control, you won't feel guilty the next day—you'll feel even more empowered to manage the crisis, says Dr. Michael Dansinger, weight-loss and nutritional consultant to *The Biggest Loser*.

Guard your sleep, too. Good health demands getting adequate sleep, and that should always top your priority list, including during a crisis. The best way to ensure that you get proper rest is to set a regular bedtime. Avoid or cut down on caffeine and alcohol—tobacco is an absolute no-no; all of these disrupt sleep patterns, making it difficult to drift off or stay there. Eating too much food close to bedtime affects many people's slumber, too.

When you remain determined not to escape

goals. Instead, get moving; start walking around your office or home, or wherever you are, and eat nutrient-rich foods that will invigorate your body's immune system and brain function, such as blueberries, fish, whole grains, and leafy green vegetables. These actions will focus your mind and give your body a much-needed boost of energy.

Your body actually becomes more resilient against the negative effects of a tough situation if you eat healthfully, take time to exercise, get adequate sleep, laugh and enjoy life, and stop trying to escape your problems through food. Healthful activities leave you feeling in better control of your life. Let's face it, no one feels in control when dig-

BIGGEST LOSER TOOLBOX

"If I'm up 5 pounds or, heaven forbid, up the ugly 10, I tell myself, 'I can't believe I've put on that much weight, ugh!' Then, I immediately replace that thought with 'The good news is that I know exactly how to take this weight off. I'm in control; I can do it in a healthy manner. It's time to get back to business.'"

—Kelly MacFarland, Season 1

into food during a crisis, you'll come out even stronger than before. Your healthy way of living will be reinforced, so you'll be able to handle any difficult situation that might arise in the future.

"Life does get in the way at times," says David Griffin, Season 4. "But with the proper motivation and a strong support network, you can handle anything."

Manage Lapses

Perhaps you lost quite a bit of weight or reached your goal, and then you slipped. Nothing is more frustrating than gaining back the weight you lost, especially after you worked so hard. The longer you wait to resume your program, the harder it is to get back on track. To keep this from happening to you, *The Biggest Loser* Online Club experts Greg Hottinger and Michael Scholtz have developed a very effective "flag system" to help you quickly recover from lapses and put them behind you.

"To make the system work, you'll need clear daily and weekly goals," Scholtz explains. "By knowing when you're on track, you'll also begin to recognize when you first start to veer off course and when you're stuck in the ditch. This system is designed to help you correct your course when you start to slide just a little and repair the damage when you've had a major crash."

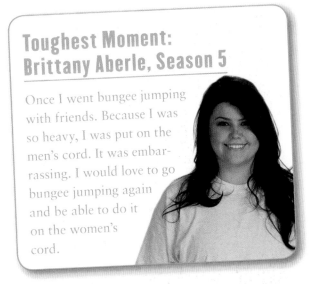

Toughest Moment: Brittany Aberle, Season 5

Once I went bungee jumping with friends. Because I was so heavy, I was put on the men's cord. It was embarrassing. I would love to go bungee jumping again and be able to do it on the women's cord.

Scholtz and Hottinger call the first part of the system "green flags." It's used to identify all the healthful activities you're doing to lose or maintain your weight. You'll want to write down these activities, which indicate that you are clearly on track. Here are some examples of green flags.

- You drink 4 glasses (48 ounces) or more of water at least 5 days a week.
- You drink 2 or fewer soft drinks a week.
- You eat 2 or 3 fruits at least 5 days a week.
- You eat 3 or more servings of vegetables 6 days a week.
- You don't skip meals.

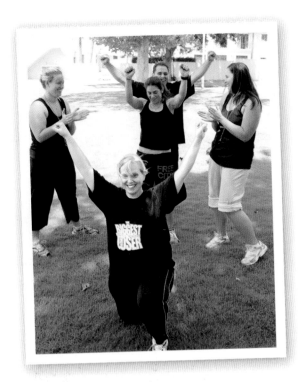

You stretch for 5 to 10 minutes after every workout.

You do exercise that makes you feel good and that you look forward to.

You listen to your body and stay injury free.

In the second part of the system are "yellow flags." These serve as warnings to help you catch yourself before you slip too far. "Relapsing into old habits is often very subtle," explains Hottinger. "Yellow flags can be indicators that you're losing motivation or have made your weight a lower priority. And in some cases, it could mean you're trying too hard, which can lead to a mental or physical breakdown." Here are examples of yellow flags.

You eat healthful snacks.

You pay attention to your food intake.

You do 2 or 3 strength-training sessions and 3 to 5 cardio sessions a week.

You burn 300 to 500 calories in each cardio session.

You keep your appointments for classes or training sessions.

You use a pedometer and reach 10,000 steps each day.

You feel tired of your food choices and notice that your meals lack variety.

You experience increased cravings for sweet or salty foods, alcohol, and other treats.

You don't get to the grocery store often enough.

You cook less often than you had been.

You miss a meal here and there and/or are snacking constantly.

- You feel more tempted by unhealthful foods at social engagements.

- You're busier than normal and have less time for food.

- After a day of eating poorly, you think that you've blown it and have lost control.

- You're not meeting your goal for daily water intake.

- You're drinking more alcohol than you'd planned.

- You rely on caffeine to get you through the day.

- You feel unmotivated and have to drag yourself to the gym.

- You cut your workouts short.

- You more often let work get in the way of exercise.

- You frequently miss a workout when it's not a planned rest day.

- It has been more than 3 days since your last workout.

- You work out at the same speed or level, but you feel like you're working harder than usual.

- You can't reach your typical speed or level during your workout.

- You work hard, but your heart rate won't rise into your training zone.

- You can't lift the same weight for the same number of reps.

"When any of these yellow flags occur, it's time to slow down a little and take stock of your schedule, your motivation, and your enjoyment," says Scholtz. "Just a small change in your routine can make the difference you need. Yellow flags are easier to correct if you catch them early."

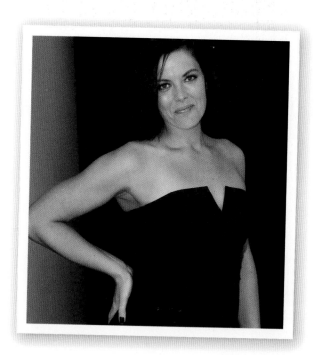

"Red flags" are the third part of the system. In the past, many of these red flags may have been everyday occurrences for you. Seeing red flags pop up on a regular basis means you're on the fast track to your old lifestyle, if you're not already there. Here are examples of red flags to watch for.

- You notice that you're not paying attention to your food and you've stopped tracking it altogether.

- You're bored with your diet and feel restricted by your food choices.

- You eat 1 or fewer fruits each day.

- You eat 2 or fewer vegetable servings each day.

- You drink less than 4 glasses (48 ounces) of water on most days.

- You drink more than 1 alcoholic drink on most days.

- You use food and/or a sugary treat as a pick-me-up.

- You stop weighing yourself so you can avoid the truth.

- You miss an entire week of exercise.

- You drop out of an exercise class or group.

- You quit meeting with your personal trainer.

- You don't renew your gym membership.

- You have a nagging injury and are not doing anything proactive to make it better.

Hottinger and Scholtz suggest that now, when your motivation is high, you make a contract with yourself and create a game plan to prevent a relapse. Here's how.

Step 1: Make a list of your yellow and red flags.

Step 2: Identify corrective steps you'll take when you see yellow or red flags.

Your plan could be as simple as:

Yellow flag: Eating zero to 2 fruits per day
Action: Go to the market, buy fruit, and track intake each day this week.

Red flag: Three unplanned missed workouts
Action: Call trainer and schedule an exercise session.

This system will help you keep careful track of your progress and avoid lapses. Don't wait another day!

The Biggest Losers in this chapter have hit rough patches, too—and they've developed great strategies for dealing with difficult times. If you adopt the ones that are helpful to you, you'll no longer be the same person who has gone off and on diets, up and down in weight, or through defeat and disillusionment. You'll start operating from a new, more powerful base of experience, one that enables you to say, "I used to have a weight problem, but now I'm a new, healthy fit person."

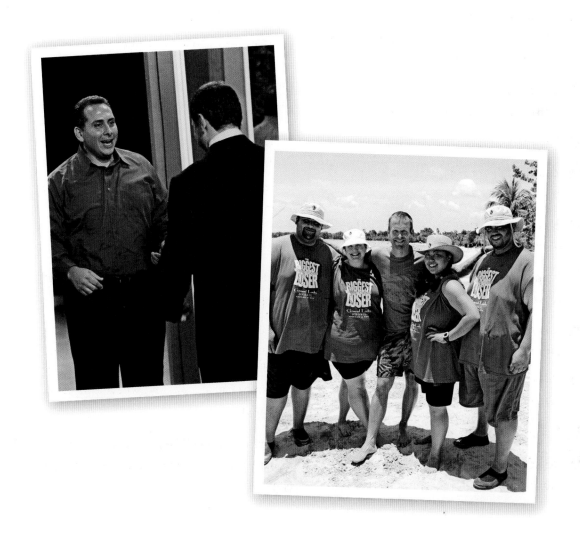

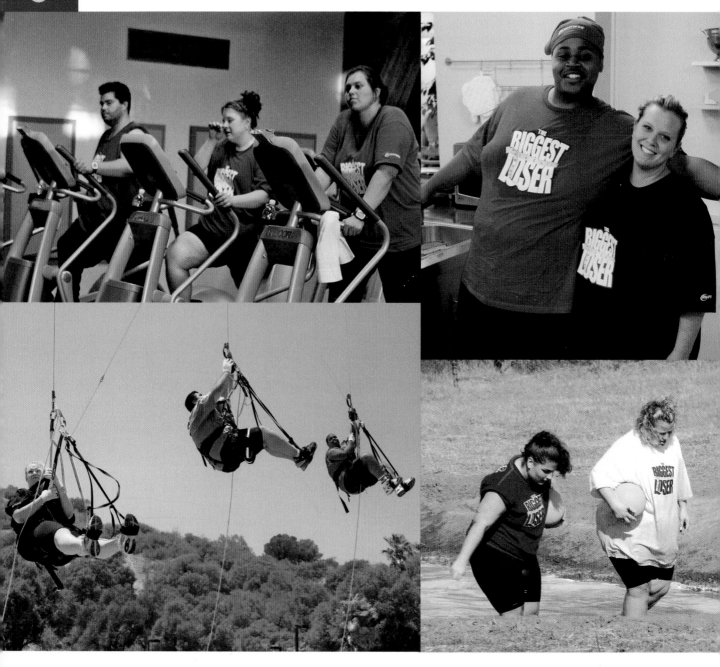

Hitting Plateaus: How to Break Through Fitness Barriers

If you've tried to get healthy before, you're probably all too familiar with one of the most frustrating aspects of weight-loss regimens: One week you diligently apply yourself to healthful eating and exercise and you're rewarded with a loss of several pounds. The next week you work just as hard, but the needle on the scale either barely moves or doesn't budge at all. As your weight loss slows to a crawl, so does your enthusiasm for your new lifestyle.

What gives?

It's the bane and downfall of many dieters: the dreaded plateau. Plateaus can occur when your daily calorie output is not much higher than your daily calorie input; or when there are major fluid shifts in your body. In other words, either you are eating too many calories and not burning enough of them, or you didn't drink enough water before your last weigh in and were dehydrated and now are appropriately replenishing your fluid stores. Your scale may fool you into mistakenly thinking your fat loss has stalled, but it *is* possible to lose fat and not lose any weight.

If the numbers on the scale are getting you down, take note of how your clothes are fitting; while you may not be losing pounds, chances are that you're still losing inches and gaining muscle tone. A pound of fat takes up a little more space than a pound of muscle. So when you lose some fat and build a little muscle, your waist, rear, and chest sizes will decrease because the muscle takes up less space. If you don't notice any difference after 3 weeks, though, it's time to rethink your diet in terms of both food choice and quantity and consider increasing the intensity of your exercise regimen.

Is there a way to break through plateaus and

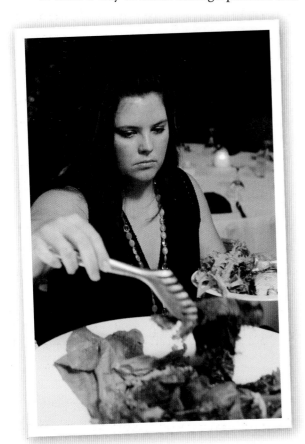

get to your goal with a minimum of frustration? You bet. That's where these plateau-busting strategies from the Biggest Losers can really help you.

Expect but Push Through Plateaus

Hollie Self, Season 4 finalist, had dropped 11 pounds at her first weigh-in, and she was thrilled. But the following week, she had shed only 2 pounds, and 3 the next. "It was discouraging to work so hard and get such limited results," she admits. But she kept going, reminding herself that numbers don't always reflect progress.

One of Hollie's strategies was to work out harder. "I needed someone to push me out of my comfort zone, to keep telling me, 'You can do more,' and my team leader and trainer, Jillian, did that for me." Hollie set new exercise goals every week. Although she hated running, one week she actually won the mini-triathlon challenge.

Double-Check Your Calorie Intake

On average, women who are on *The Biggest Loser* diet consume between 1,100 and 1,500 calories a day; men, between 1,500 and 2,300. If you're not sure whether you're on target, record the foods you eat and when you eat them for 3 days and be sure

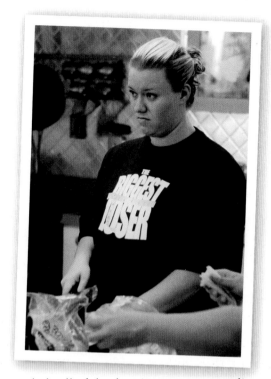

to include all of the dressings, sauces, condiments, and other "extras" you use to flavor your meal. *The Biggest Loser Complete Calorie Counter* lists calories for more than 5,000 foods and can be a powerful tool to help you tally up your calories.

If you have plateaued, there is a good chance you're eating too many calories. Research shows that dieters often underreport their caloric intake and overreport how much they're working out. In a study reported in *The New England Journal of Medicine,* researchers looked at a group of obese men and women who were having trouble losing weight. Was it their metabolism? Was it genetics?

Neither. They were eating more than they thought they were and exercising less than they figured. Sometimes it's easy to let a few hundred calories sneak into your diet, and even that small amount can prevent weight loss. It could be as simple as forgetting to order skim milk in your daily latte or adding extra condiments to your favorite sandwich. Every extra calorie adds up, so weigh and measure everything. Examine your food journal to make sure you're not eating processed foods, either. These can spike your diet with unwanted calories. Review every aspect of your program: Have you been eating out? Restaurant food is laden with hidden calories that may disrupt your steady progress. Depending on what your food journal reveals, you may need to scale back your portions or make better food choices. Natural, unprocessed foods are bursting with nutrients, each put to use in building and healing the body, while processed foods can be nutritionally bankrupt and associated with various health problems. It's always important to include variety in your diet, though, in order to ensure that your body is

BIGGEST LOSER TOOLBOX

"If you plateau, don't panic. It's your body getting used to your new size."
—Kelly Fields, Season 5

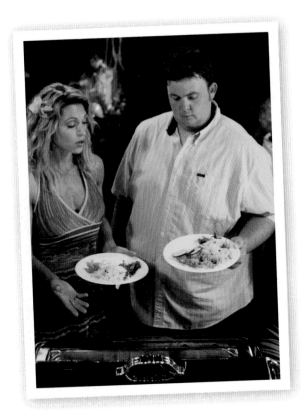

Adjust Your Calories

One change to consider is adjusting your caloric intake slightly. Your initial estimate of your true caloric needs may have been too high, resulting in less weight loss than you'd hoped for. Also, as you bid farewell to those pounds and inches, your calorie requirement may drop slightly, according to Dr. Michael Dansinger, weight-loss and nutritional consultant to *The Biggest Loser*. Here's why: for every pound of fat you lose, you decrease the num-

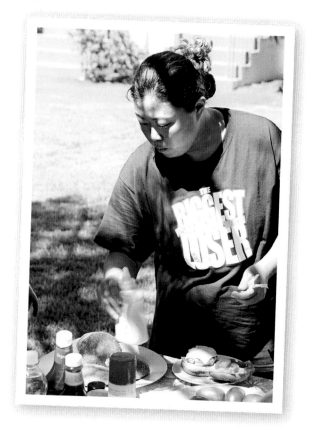

getting all the essential nutrients for good health.

"As you go through this analysis, be 100 percent honest," recommends Season 4's David Griffin. "If you keep doing the right thing, the scale will catch up."

"When people plateau, there are options," adds Kae Whang, Season 4. "First, you have to monitor whether you're doing something that brought on the plateau. Then you have to make adjustments or get back on track. Believe me, I know. Your body will respond when you make changes!"

ber of calories you expend each day by about 10. That's roughly the number of calories that were required to keep that fat at body temperature, move it around, and support its metabolic needs. So if you shed 10 pounds of fat, you could burn about 100 fewer calories each day. On the other hand, losing weight tends to boost your mood and give you more energy, so you may find yourself burning some extra calories with all of that new-found energy. In any case, when it's time for you to adjust your calories, there are four easy, near-automatic ways to do it if you are following *The Biggest Loser* diet.

1. Cut your calories from the optional 200-calorie budget allowed on the diet.

2. Replace your whole-grain servings with vegetables.

3. Choose lower-calorie, nonmeat proteins, such as low-fat yogurt, egg whites, and soy.

4. Reduce one fruit serving in favor of one more vegetable serving.

BIGGEST LOSER TOOLBOX

"If you tend to overeat or oversnack in front of the television, make it a rule in your house to always eat in the dining room while seated at the table."

—Pam Smith, Season 3

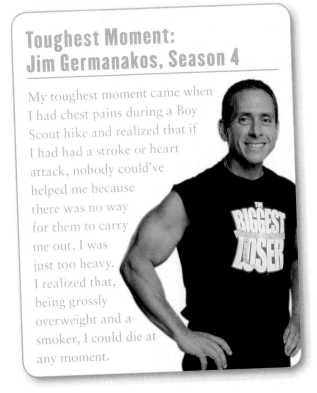

Toughest Moment: Jim Germanakos, Season 4

My toughest moment came when I had chest pains during a Boy Scout hike and realized that if I had had a stroke or heart attack, nobody could've helped me because there was no way for them to carry me out. I was just too heavy. I realized that, being grossly overweight and a smoker, I could die at any moment.

Just don't get discouraged! You'll continue losing on *The Biggest Loser* diet because it keeps your calorie, carb, and fat intakes in check. The worst thing you can do when you are frustrated by hitting a plateau is to deviate from what's been working for you so far.

Get Enough Protein Each Day

Protein is to your body what a wooden frame is to your house. Nutritionally, it is a basic, important building block in your body, essential to optimal health because of its role in supporting cell growth and maintenance. Your body breaks down protein from food into nutrient fragments called amino acids and reshuffles them into new proteins to build new tissues and repair damaged tissues, including body-firming muscle. Protein also keeps your immune system functioning up to par, helps carry nutrients throughout the body, and is involved in important enzymatic reactions such as digestion.

Adds *Biggest Loser* nutritionist Cheryl Forberg, RD: "Protein helps slow the release of blood sugar, promoting fullness and sustained energy, which allows you to exercise more." If you don't get enough protein, your body can start breaking down muscle tissue. Consequently, you may lose calorie-burning muscle, which can sabotage your fat-loss efforts.

Best Moment: Maggie King, Season 5

I had resigned myself to being fat for the rest of my life. Then I was selected for *The Biggest Loser*, and I realized I don't have to be fat forever. I can do this.

The Biggest Loser diet recommends having three 8-ounce (1 cup) portions of protein-rich foods each day. If your fat loss has plateaued and you're doing everything else right, bump up your protein intake slightly in exchange for other calories in your budget. Proteins included in *The Biggest Loser* diet include fish, lean meats, poultry, eggs, soy foods, legumes, and reduced-fat dairy products. It's best to eat some protein with each meal so your body can use it throughout the day.

Water Your Body

The general rule of thumb for water intake while losing weight is to drink at least 6 glasses of pure water daily. At times on *The Biggest Loser*, the contestants have been threatened with penalties if they become dehydrated. Water is that important!

"Marty and I have a case of bottled water in our car at all times," says Amy Hildreth, Season 3. "You need to stay hydrated."

If you feel thirsty, chances are you're already mildly dehydrated. In fact, people who exercise regularly can get mildly dehydrated even before their body has a chance to warn them by feeling thirsty. One symptom to look out for is fatigue. Dehydration might make you feel tired, since water is involved in energy-producing processes in the body. Water also dissolves vitamins, minerals, proteins, glucose, and other nutrients and carries them

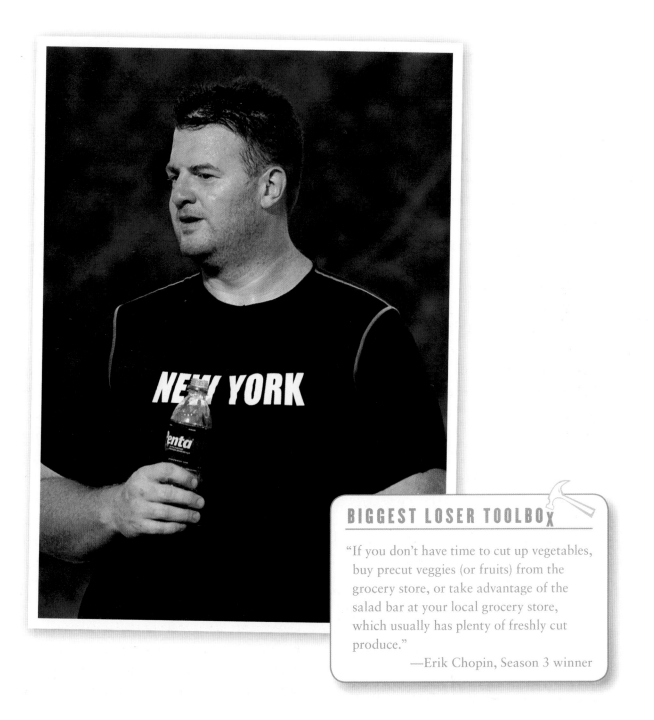

BIGGEST LOSER TOOLBOX

"If you don't have time to cut up vegetables, buy precut veggies (or fruits) from the grocery store, or take advantage of the salad bar at your local grocery store, which usually has plenty of freshly cut produce."

—Erik Chopin, Season 3 winner

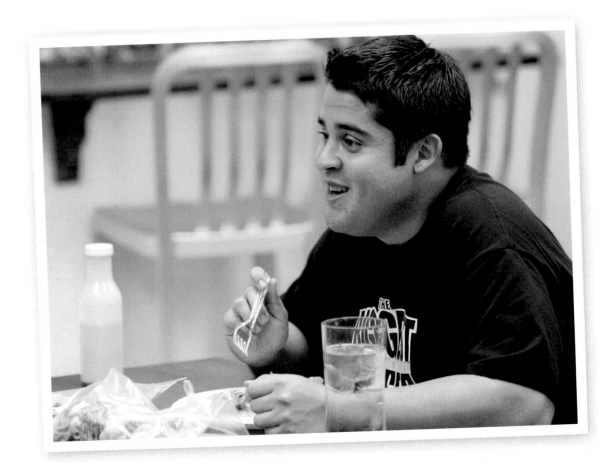

to your cells, while simultaneously washing away waste products.

Another way to check how well you've watered your body is by checking the color of your urine. If it's pale yellow, you're well hydrated; if it's on the dark side, you might be dehydrated. Perfectly clear urine indicates water overload and implies you can probably cut down on your fluid intake.

Also, the more you exercise, the more water your body will require to replenish what is lost through sweating. Try to drink about 8 ounces of water 1 hour before you exercise (if you drink it immediately before exercising, you may end up with a painful cramp), sip water or a low-calorie sports drink while you work out, and have another glass or two after you finish your cooldown. If you get bored with the taste of water, try flavoring a pitcher or bottle of plain water with herbs like mint or basil, or slices of citrus fruits or cucumber. You'll create "spa water" in no time!

Watch Your Salt Intake

While it's always important to get enough water-based fluids, salt intake is considerably trickier. The average American who doesn't exercise consumes excess salt and is at risk for fluid retention and hypertension. On the other hand, regular exercisers lose salt in their sweat. In fact, some who sweat heavily and eat low-calorie, high fruit, vegetable, and lean protein diets actually need to *add* salt to their food. Bottom line, once you start a daily exercise program, you no longer have to check the labels of foods for their salt contents or

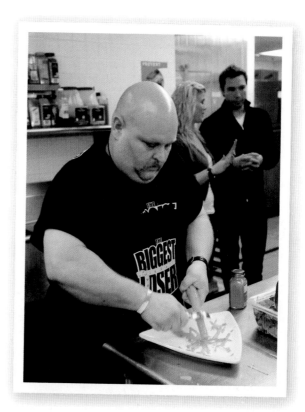

The Biggest Loser Online Club Profile: Cindy Beier

Starting weight: 223.5 • Current weight: 144 • Goal weight: 135

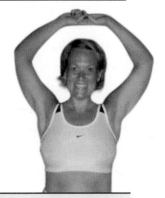

Cindy never successfully lost weight until she joined *The Biggest Loser* Online Club. "I've started a diet almost every week of my life but usually ended up quitting within the day, determined to start the following Monday. I'd eat as much as I could during that week because 'I was never going to have these foods again.' But the Club got me serious about losing weight." Cindy loves the menu plans and the recipes and uses *The Biggest Loser* Diet to overcome plateaus and get back on track if she falls victim to emotional eating.

"I have energy like never before," she says. "I'm a new person."

Change your life today! Log on to www.biggestloserclub.com and get started.

select only the low-salt or salt-free versions (like you did when you were a couch potato). You're sweating out that salt now!

Revamp Your Exercise Program

As was discussed earlier in this book, it's a good idea to change your routine and introduce new activities and exercises into your workout to con-

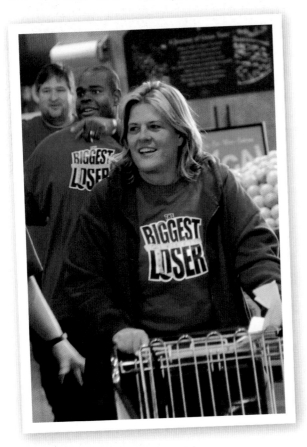

dition as many muscles as possible and to keep your mind from getting bored. Try learning a new sport, like racquetball or boxing, or take a dance class. You could change your strength-training program by alternating between doing fewer reps with heavy weights one week and more reps with lighter weights the next. Or take up circuit training, a metabolism booster that is recommended in *The Biggest Loser Fitness Program*. Circuit training combines cardio training with strength training and is a terrific fat burner. Another option is to try interval training, a method in which you alternate high-intensity training with lower-intensity training. For example, you might run or jog at a speed that is comfortable for you for 8 minutes (low-intensity training) and then run at a speed that challenges you for 2 minutes (high-intensity training), and continue alternating for the duration of your workout.

"My routine changes about every 2 to 3 months as I try to find the perfect workout for weight maintenance," explains Pete Thomas, Season 2, who is maintaining a 160-pound weight loss. "I believe you should stick with a routine for at least 8 weeks to properly assess its effectiveness." Periodically, Pete returns to "the exercise basics"—a full-body strength-training program three times a week combined with 1 hour of medium-intensity cardio (performed at at least 75 percent of his maximum heart rate) three times a week.

Season 3's Biggest Loser, Erik Chopin, has a similar strategy. "If the scale isn't giving me a good number, I look at what I'm doing, and maybe I'll

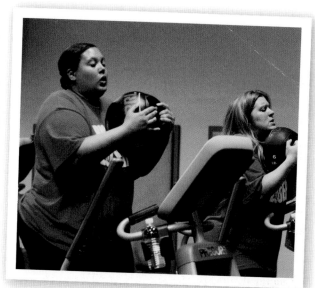

Consider a Personal Trainer

To blast through that plateau, maybe you need a trainer to nudge you a little harder in your workouts. If that's an option for you, Michael Scholtz, *Biggest Loser* Club fitness expert, suggests that you interview a few different trainers before you sign up for anything. It's important to find the right person to help you achieve your goals. Be sure to ask:

- If they are certified, and by what organization
- If they have liability insurance and with whom
- What their business practices are in regard to cancellations and billing
- If they plan to document your medical history and progress
- How much they charge and how (by the session? by the hour?)
- Where does the trainer work and does that location work for you? Consider where you'd be most comfortable—at a gym? At home?

It's also a good idea to ask for references from other clients. In the end, Scholtz says one of the most important qualities in a potential trainer is that they are "someone you can work with." Make sure the person you have in mind subscribes to a fitness philosophy similar to yours, clearly understands your goals, and seems focused on your success. You should look forward to time with your trainer—not dread it!

switch up my routine a little bit. Change can be invigorating. If one week I see my weight slowly creeping up, that's a message to me to change my workout the next week."

Andrea Overstreet, Season 2, agrees—and puts a positive spin on plateaus. "Plateaus are a signal to me that my body is getting used to my routine or my diet, and that I need to change something up. So instead of going to the gym, I might go running, swimming, or mountain biking."

Don't Neglect Strength Training

Sometimes we get so preoccupied with cardio maximum-heart-rate zones and feeling the endorphin rush that we forget how important it is to build muscle. Strength training burns extra fat by creating metabolically active muscle tissue. (Fat tissue is less metabolically active and does not burn as many calories.) Muscle tissue burns fat,

and the more muscle you have, the more calories you burn—even when you're at rest. In other words, building muscle increases your resting metabolic rate. Strength training also helps your metabolism stay charged up long after your workout ends. Even as few as three 30-minute sessions a week can make a difference. And you don't need an expensive gym membership, either. A stability ball, resistance bands, and some free weights are all you need to get started.

Rethink Your Goal Weight

If you've plateaued at a weight that's near your goal, it may be that your body has already reached its healthy, natural weight and has settled in the spot where it is supposed to be. "I experienced a plateau around 140 pounds," comments Kae Whang, Season 4. "At first I couldn't understand it, but now I see that my body was telling me, 'This is your healthy weight now,' and it was time to work on maintenance."

Isabeau Miller, Season 4 finalist, adds that many people pick goal weights that sound good but may not be realistic for them. "You might have to reevaluate your own goals and see if they are reasonable or if they're just society's standards or someone else's standards for you. It's really hard to tune out the pressure from other

---

BIGGEST LOSER TOOLBOX

"Hang your goal outfit—a bikini, suit, cocktail dress, or skinny pants—on a door handle or somewhere visible—as a reminder of what you will accomplish."
—Hollie Self, Season 4

people, but ultimately you're the one you have to live with, and if you are happy with yourself, then no one else really matters."

Most people are inclined to think of a plateau as a negative, but not Season 4's Neil Tejwani. "Yes, plateaus are discouraging, but your body's not letting go of a few extra pounds is not necessarily a bad thing. It's all part of the journey you're taking to better health."

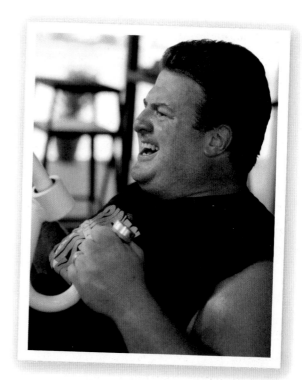

Use Your Mantra

Since Season 2, contestants have been using mantras—positive affirmations to help them get over negative head trips and keep their attention centered

---

Biggest Loser Mantras

These are some of the mantras used by Season 4 contestants to help them through plateaus and keep them focused on their goals.

Kae Whang: To visit my family

David Griffin: For the loves of my life

Hollie Self: To practice what I preach

Bill Germankos: To become half the man so I can be twice the man

Isabeau Miller: To be a rock star

Neil Tejwani: To be a stallion

Julie Hadden: To finish what I started for once

Jim Germanakos: To be here for me, for them, forever

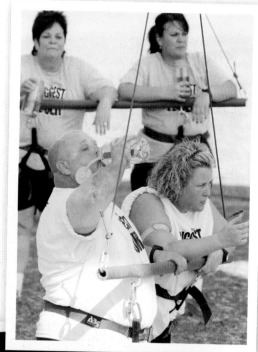

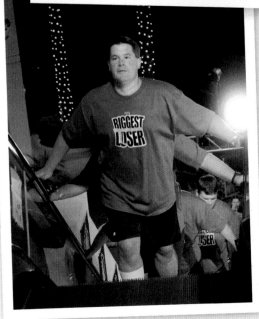

and focused on their goals. A mantra comes in handy when you're wrestling with a plateau and struggling with moments of doubt. Finding a mantra worked for Season 4's Isabeau Miller. "When I started questioning my ability to keep losing weight, I would remember the last thing my parents said before I left for the show: 'Never, ever give up.'" The more you use your mantra, the more easily it will become part of your positive thought process and a vehicle to help you overcome plateaus.

Be Patient

If you're overly anxious, your body might increase its output of cortisol, a stress hormone that, when chronically elevated, might promote fat gain, especially around the waist. Exercise can mitigate this problem, as can getting adequate sleep, meditating, and doing relaxation exercises.

"Just keep in mind that the body does not lose weight in a consistent manner. It is normal to lose during one week, plateau during another, and then lose weight again," explains Dr. Michael Dansinger, weight-loss and nutritional consultant to *The Biggest Loser.* Be patient, and focus on what you *can* control. Stay on track with your diet and work hard to meet your exercise goals. If you do these things regularly, you will lose weight. It's as simple as that.

Keep in mind, too, that the Biggest Losers devote all of their time to dieting and exercising while they're at the ranch, which is how they achieve the double-digit weight losses you see on the show. That won't happen under normal circumstances, so don't compare your numbers to what you view on the screen. You're doing great if you're losing up to 2 pounds a week, on average (depending on your metabolism, daily calorie burn, and starting weight).

Think of your progress in terms of Aesop's fable about the tortoise and the hare. The slow but steady tortoise wins the race, even though his opponent, the hare, is a faster sprinter. You didn't gain all the weight you hope to lose overnight, and you're not going to lose it that fast, either. Keep in mind that losing weight at the rate of 1 to 2 pounds per week adds up to 50 to 100 pounds in just a year!

Measure Success in Other Ways

When Dr. Robert Huizenga took the Season 5 cast members on a tour of the morgue, he wanted to drive home the fact that their health was in jeopardy—and that if they didn't change, they could wind up there. "This tour gave them something else besides a lower weight to shoot for—their lifelong health," he says.

Success is not only quantified by scales or the

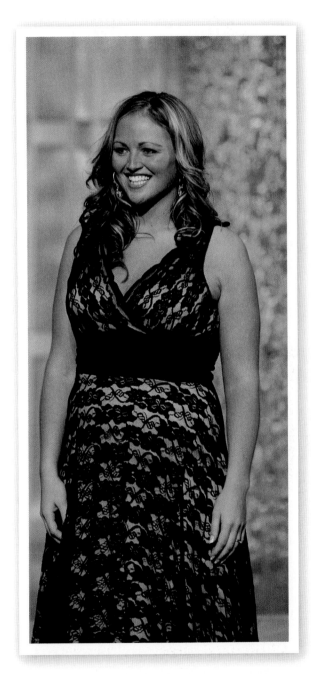

reflection in the mirror, it is also measured by your physical and mental health. If you committed yourself to leading a healthful lifestyle, chances are you're feeling energetic and positive. It's hard not to notice that! Check in with yourself, physically and emotionally, and note the positive changes in your mental outlook. Or maybe the positive changes you've made are already reflected in your physical health. When Biggest Loser Erik Chopin joined Season 3 as the biggest guy there, he was also diagnosed with some big health problems: type 2 diabetes, high blood pressure, and high cholesterol. "When I found out that I was on my way to a heart attack, I was shocked. I wanted to survive and be healthy for my wife and kids," he says. Committing to a healthy lifestyle has put his health problems into remission—without medication, which is nothing short of miraculous! (If you have similar problems or issues, always consult your physician about your medications and dosages, as well as your diet and exercise program; don't make changes on your own.)

To assess your progress and confirm that you're losing fat, not lean tissue, you may also want to periodically check your body composition. Unfortunately, the commonly available bioelectrical impedance (BIA) bathroom scales you can buy at local stores are sometimes inaccurate, especially in the face of weight loss or dehydration. When indicated, your doctor or trainer can refer you to the nearest Bod Pod or underwater weighting site for more reliable body fat determinations.

"I think people are too obsessed with their weight on the scale instead of how clothes fit them, or other measures of success," says Kae Whang, Season 4. "If you're feeling energized, happy, and healthy, these are all major life improvements that deserve a celebration—regardless of what the scale shows."

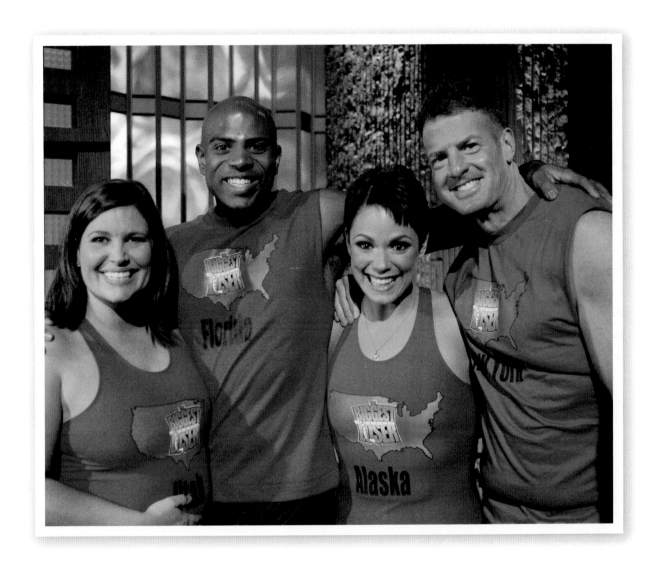

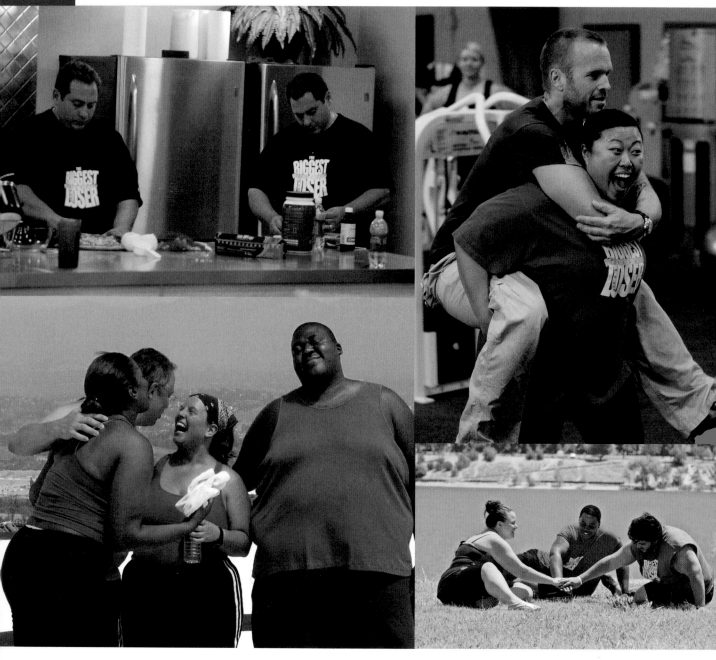

Support or Sabotage? The Powerful Influence of Family and Friends

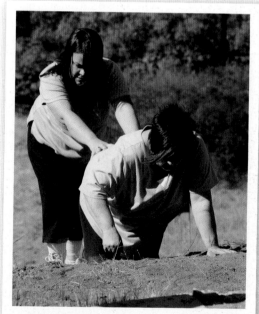

It could be your spouse, your mother, your best friend. They know you're on a plan to eat right and exercise regularly. You've told them a million times. But then comes the giant birthday cake ("It's a special occasion!"), the pizza with everything on it ("It's a treat—just this once!"), the invitation to an all-you-can-eat pancake breakfast ("Your whole family will be there!"). How can you stick to your commitment when you're surrounded by people who—knowingly or unknowingly—are undermining your efforts?

The answer is straightforward: Surround yourself with people who are supportive.

Talk to any cast member from any season, and each will tell you how vital it is to be supported by loved ones while you're on your weight-loss regimen—and after. David Griffin's wife quit her job in medical sales, took the reins of the family farm, and handled everything while he was at the ranch losing weight during Season 4. "Now that I'm back home, she makes sure I can get to the gym. She monitors my nutrition. From time to time, she'll say, 'Should you be eating this late at night?' My whole family is involved. My kids even hid their Halloween candy from me!"

Bette-Sue Burklund auditioned for *The Biggest Loser* to support her daughter, Ali Vincent. They were partners in Season 5.

Andrea Overstreet, Season 2, says her husband has always told her she is beautiful, no matter how much she weighs. "He's amazing. Without his support, I'm not sure I'd do as well. You need someone who loves you for you."

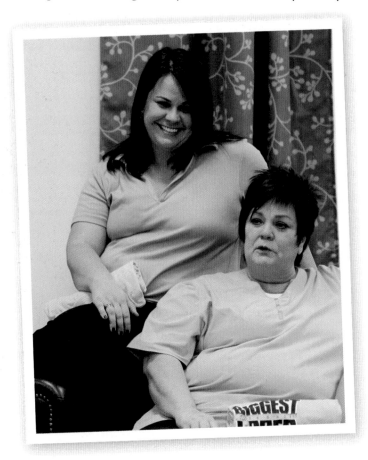

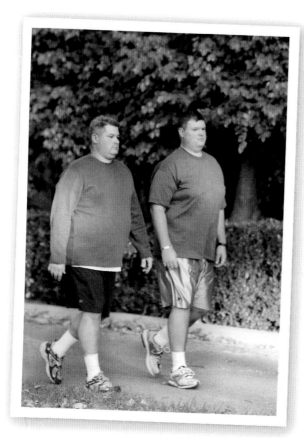

BIGGEST LOSER TOOLBOX

"I wake up every morning and tell myself, 'This is a new day for me to change my life and make myself a better person than I was yesterday.'"

—Dan Evans, Season 5

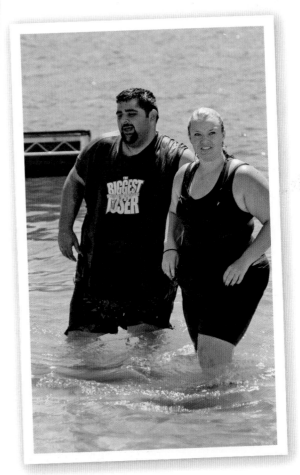

At the ranch during Season 5, Mark Kruger leaned on his brother and *Biggest Loser* partner, Jay. They are supporting each other back home, too. "If I have a moment of weakness, it's a real easy phone call to Jay. Plus, we see each other every day since we work for the same company."

When she notices that her weight has started climbing uncomfortably high, Kelly MacFarland, Season 1, huddles with her trainers, coaches, and others she enlisted for "Team Kelly." "I let them know what the scoop is—that I'm up 5 or 10 pounds. So, give me some extra work!"

Season 2's Pete Thomas believes that you must have a team around you if you're going to lose weight successfully. "My wife is my teammate. While I was at the ranch, she lost 70 pounds. Today, we're helping each other live a healthy lifestyle. I credit her with helping me keep my weight off."

Kae Whang, Season 4, and her husband have overhauled their leisure time to be more active. "Where once we used to veg out in the sun on vacations, now we've decided to go skiing in the Alps or try some extreme sports in New Zealand. He's very supportive and excited about taking active vacations, too."

Husband-and-wife Biggest Losers Matt Hoover and Suzy Preston, Season 2, say the great-

est thing about their marriage is open communication. One thing they're very honest about with one another is food. Matt knows that chips and salsa are a trigger for Suzy, so he does not bring them into the house. "When you love someone," he emphasizes, "that's what you do." "We encourage each other," Suzy adds, "and never set each other up to fail."

And if one wants to call out the other about a diet slipup? "Just be honest," Suzy advises, "not accusatory."

"We have to watch our food forever," Matt says. "I could end up on *Biggest Loser* 6 if I don't watch it!"

Whether it's your neighbor who shows up every morning to walk with you, a spouse who encourages you to keep going when you've hit a plateau, or a mother-in-law who cooks a special plate for you at a family dinner, studies reveal that a support network boosts your ability to make the lifestyle changes necessary to lose weight and keep it off.

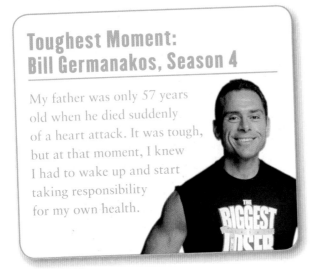

Toughest Moment:
Bill Germanakos, Season 4

My father was only 57 years old when he died suddenly of a heart attack. It was tough, but at that moment, I knew I had to wake up and start taking responsibility for my own health.

Dealing with Saboteurs

Season 3 winner Erik Chopin, who registered the most dramatic weight loss in the history of the show, admits that he's a former diet saboteur. He would take home junk foods like pizza and ice cream to share with his wife, Michele. "I dragged her down with me," he says. "It was like having a partner in crime." But she was the first to quit their unhealthy lifestyle, joining a gym even before Erik made the final cut for *The Biggest Loser*. While he was away at the ranch, she ran the family business (which, just to make things even harder, was a deli!), cared for their two daughters—and, remarkably, lost 60 pounds.

Often, you'll have friends or relatives who insist that you sample their famous apple pie or who act hurt when you refuse a second helping at the dinner table. They probably aren't deliberately trying to interfere with your weight loss. Usually these people have good intentions, but they don't fully understand what's at stake for you (those extra 400 calories mean squeezing in an extra trip to the gym) or just how hard it is to make progress. While the cause of these actions might be genuine concern for your happiness and contentment, the effect is almost always destructive.

Other times, you'll find yourself confronted by people who—motivated by envy or their own

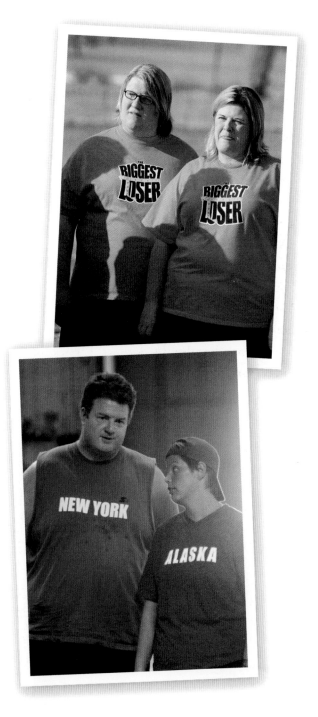

insecurities—don't want you to get thin, and repeatedly try to scuttle your diet. For example, if you and your best friend were both heavy and that fact served as a bond for your friendship, he or she might feel threatened by your weight loss and jealous of your success. Those feelings can drive a wedge of resentment into your relationship—especially if your friend intentionally tries to ruin your progress.

Why would anyone act like this?

"Basically, the people in our lives learn to expect and rely on us to be who we have always been," explains Alexa Altman, the psychologist for *The Biggest Loser*. "This is an important concept to acknowledge as you continue to forge ahead with your weight loss, because your social environment can further reinforce or sabotage your efforts."

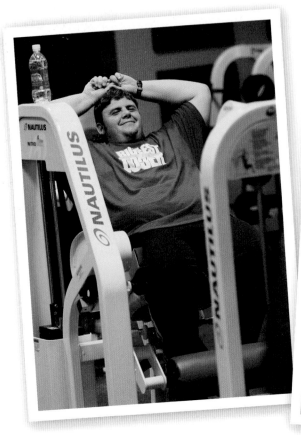

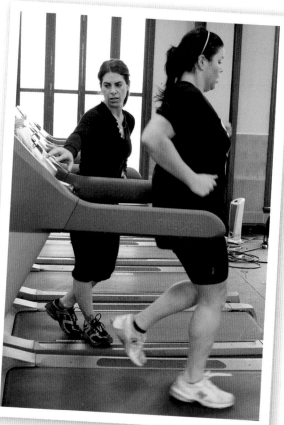

Altman suggests identifying, preparing for, and protecting yourself from those in your environment who either deliberately or innocently may be jeopardizing your health and well-being. Begin by asking yourself some basic questions to identify who is negatively impacting your weight-loss efforts. After each question, write the initials of the person or people.

☐ Who refuses to eat with me at the healthier restaurants that I suggest?_____

☐ Who insists that we go to fast-food restaurants and buffets?_____

☐ Who discounts or laughs at my efforts to lose weight?_____

☐ Who brings junk food into my home or to my desk at work?_____

☐ Who complains about the time I take to cook or exercise?_____

☐ Who tells me I "don't need to be on a diet" when I know that I do?_____

☐ Who makes me feel singled out when I don't want to eat sweets or overindulge with a group?_____

If a set of initials is next to each question or the same person plays many of these roles, you have to protect yourself. There is a saboteur lurking.

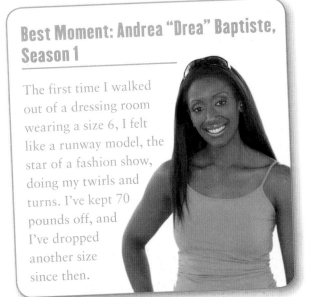

Best Moment: Andrea "Drea" Baptiste, Season 1

The first time I walked out of a dressing room wearing a size 6, I felt like a runway model, the star of a fashion show, doing my twirls and turns. I've kept 70 pounds off, and I've dropped another size since then.

Altman says it is critical to set limits or use boundaries to protect yourself from such people, both emotionally and physically. "We have all had the experience of someone getting a little too close and bumping up against our physical boundary or personal space," she explains. "Our body usually lets us know when our boundary is being violated: we get uncomfortable and we want to move away.

BIGGEST LOSER TOOLBOX

"Tell your friends and family that you're on the *Biggest Loser* food plan and that you need their support!"
—Trent Patterson, Season 5

Emotional boundaries are similar in that they also protect us from unwanted intrusion. When we have good boundaries, there is often a sense of feeling protected or safe in the world."

When it comes to dealing with saboteurs, you can set a "good" boundary by being assertive and expressing what you want or need—in other words, by standing up for yourself. This not the same as being aggressive, which means attacking people or pushing them around. Being assertive is

The Biggest Loser Online Club Profile: **Michelle Best**

Starting weight: 313 • Current weight: 263 • Goal weight: 130

Support has been vital in Michelle's success and she found it in several corners of her life. For starters, she and her husband decided to make a health transformation together. She would lose weight, and he would quit smoking.

Michelle immediately became a member of *The Biggest Loser* Online Club. "I knew deep down, I really needed to lose this weight and I was hoping this would finally be the time and the Club would be my miracle."

What Michelle likes best about the Club is the community that pulls together to support and encourage one another. "For me, that has been the drive behind my success. I could not have had this success without meeting the friends that I have online."

In fact, Michelle built support right away. "When I first started *The Biggest Loser* Online Club, I started my own support group. We're called the 'Healthy Hotties.' We post daily about our successes, struggles, what we eat, recipes, etc. We hold each other accountable for what we are doing and we post if we are having a hard time. I'm also in 3 challenge groups. They really help me to stay accountable for the calories, water, and exercise. People at work have already started to notice my success and ask me how much I've lost. One coworker even signed up for Club herself!"

Michelle also advises looking to club members for advice. "They are always there to help you with something you are not sure about or are having trouble with."

Change your life today! Log on to www.biggestloserclub.com and get started.

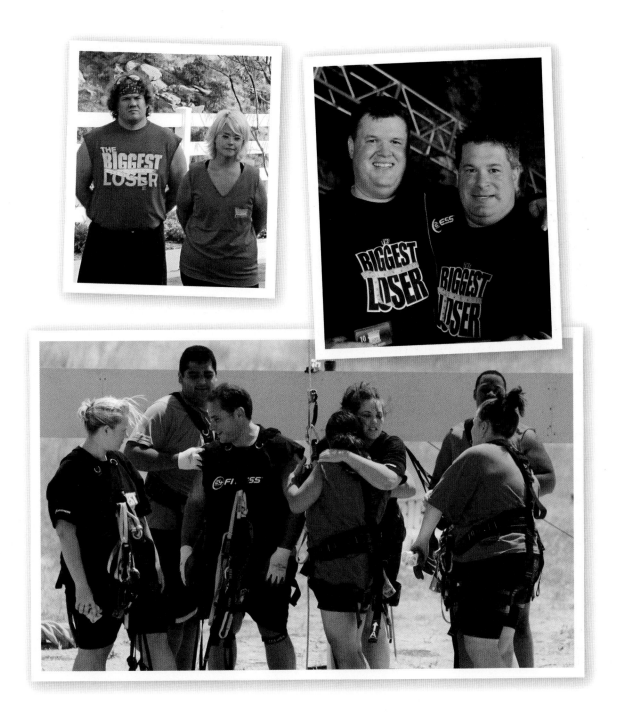

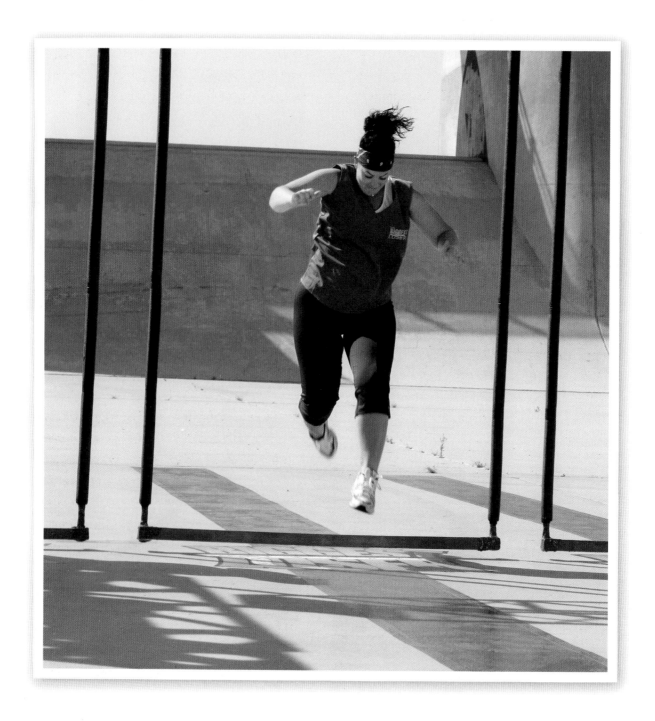

a weight-control skill, one that's as important as counting calories or becoming more physically active. Standing up for yourself can be done tactfully, without endangering relationships or hurting feelings, and communicated in a way that wins people over.

Ask people to help you in small ways—by reminding you of your goals when you feel weak, not tempting you by eating problem foods in front of you, or supporting you during stressful moments when depending on food is not an option. Be specific in telling them what you need: "It would help me if you don't get me a birthday cake this year," for example. Also, be clear about what things might annoy you, such as your spouse policing you with comments like "Is that on your diet?"

Andrea Overstreet, Season 2, believes that it is helpful to plan ahead if you know you might be

around saboteurs. "If I'm trying to eat healthy or shed a few pounds but I'm invited to an event where all the wrong foods will be served, I'll ask permission to bring some of my own food. Or I'll politely explain to the hostess my reasons for not eating certain foods."

Sometimes you may have to reevaluate your relationships and avoid certain people, at least for a while, if they continue to hamper your program. This was a choice Andrea "Drea" Baptiste, Season 1, had to make. "I had some unsupportive people in my life who were like poison. I had to let them go so that I could maintain my healthy lifestyle."

Turn Saboteurs into Supporters

Learn how to ask for and negotiate support, rather than demanding it, from the people in your life who are willing to help. Avoid vague, general requests such as "I'd like you to be more supportive." It is unfair to others to ask for help and expect them to know automatically and precisely how to respond. So be specific here, too. For example, "Would you be willing to snack in the kitchen rather than in the den, in front of me?" is a very specific request.

Another approach might be to ask a reluctant spouse, friend, or relative to actually participate in your program in a small way. Try inviting him or

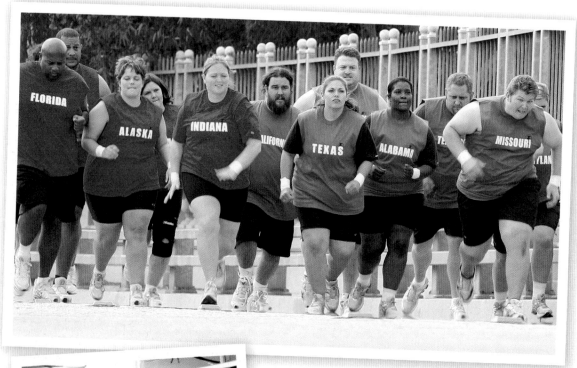

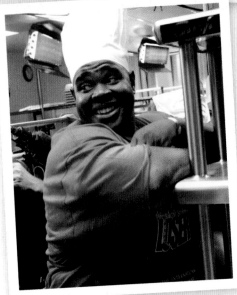

her to a fun exercise class with you, or cook a healthy meal from your new repertoire for the two of you. Your conversation with your spouse might go something like this: "I want to spend more time with you because I love being together. Let's try an exercise program together, just for 2 weeks, to see how we like it. Wouldn't that be a great way to spend time together?" To a friend or relative, you might say, "I'd like to stay in touch with you more often. Why don't we go bicycling around the neighborhood, to keep each other motivated?"

If they make these small changes, they will help you stick with your program. Researchers who studied a group of married people who began a yearlong exercise program found that only 6 percent of those who worked out together dropped out, compared to 43 percent of those who exercised solo, according to the results published in *The Journal of Sports Medicine and Physical Fitness.*

Sharing the fitness experience gives you both something new to do and something new to talk about. At the end of the trial period, as a sign of appreciation, give your partner some type of healthful gift, such as a new pair of sneakers or a gift certificate for a session with a trainer. By that time, hopefully, your partner will want to join you in continuing this powerful lifestyle.

Suzy Preston, a Season 2 finalist, says dealing with people boils down to honesty. "If you have a spouse who is thin, have a heart-to-heart talk with him or her and explain your struggles. Someone who doesn't have a weight problem may not under-

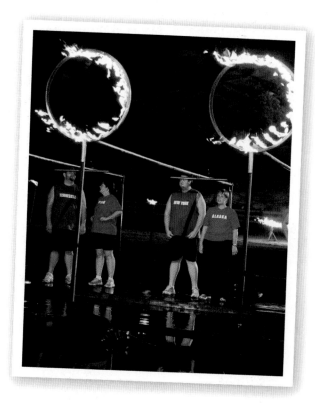

stand how tempting it is to be around junk. Say, for instance, 'When you keep ice cream in the freezer, I'm tempted to eat it, and when I do, I gain weight and feel bad about it. It would really help me if you would be willing to buy low-fat frozen yogurt, instead.'"

While she was pregnant with her son, Suzy gained some "baby weight." She had to tell her friends that she and Matt couldn't go out to dinner just yet because they were both working on their weight. Instead, they invited friends over to their

BIGGEST LOSER TOOLBOX

"If you think you can't get to the gym because you need a babysitter, think again. A lot of gyms have babysitting services on site so parents can work out."

—Suzy Preston, Season 2

house for dinner and cooked a healthy meal to enjoy.

If your spouse (or kids) insists on eating fattening foods or desserts, work around it. You can still make your family's favorite foods and simply adjust your own portions. "Or fill your plate with veggies, and serve high-calorie foods like macaroni and cheese as side dishes or occasional treats," says Jackie Evans, Season 5.

Be patient with others in their attempts to help you. Just as you may experience setbacks, others may occasionally lapse into using previously unsupportive tactics. Remember that they are learning, too. Their habits may be just as hard to change as your own, and any long-term change requires time, patience, and effort.

In the end, your commitment to health can inspire the people you love to improve their own lives. Keep your commitment to developing a fit lifestyle. If your spouse or loved ones see consistency in your life, they're more likely to follow in your footsteps.

BIGGEST LOSER TOOLBOX

"If support isn't readily available at first, keep this book handy and use us as your support group to inspire you."
—Bill Germanakos, Season 4

Build Your Team

One big reason cast members are so successful on the show is the support they receive from the enormous team of trainers, physicians, and dietitians—not to mention the other contestants—at the ranch, who are there every day to offer guidance and moral support. But you can build your own winning team right at home. The first step is to recognize who would make the best team members. People can provide support in many different ways. Some people are good at giving advice and listening to you without judging. There are others with whom you can share your trials and triumphs because you're both trying to lose weight. These people can act as sounding boards or provide a safe place to put aside masks and express honest feelings. Sometimes you may want someone to give you practical support, such as wanting a spouse to help out with extra chores while you cook dinner or a parent to watch your children while you go to the gym.

Connecting with like-minded people who encourage you to reach your goals not only provides valuable support, it will also give you a network of people who hold you accountable for meeting the targets you've set. Maybe you need a buddy who can exercise or diet with you. When Kae Whang, Season 4, got home, her first step was to hook up with a weight-training buddy who's

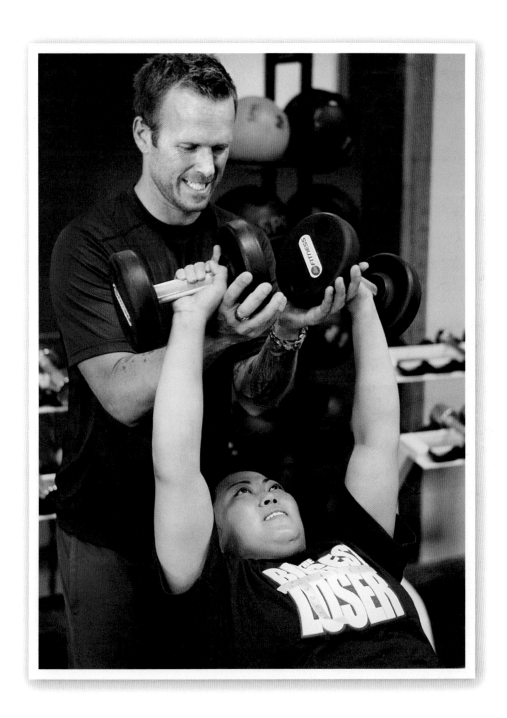

just as motivating as her on-the-set trainer, Bob Harper. "Bob got to know each of us personally, but in the gym, he was dead serious. I wanted to find someone just like that," she says. Some of us need a "cheerleader" to provide encouragement and inspiration so we can maintain our focus, or a technical person with real expertise, such as a personal trainer, dietitian, or physician.

Any one of these people might serve as a mentor with whom you can review your progress weekly—and it just might accelerate your weight loss. In one study, people who cut their calorie intake, exercised, and checked in with another person about their progress lost almost twice as much weight as those who didn't have a mentor.

Think about the people in your life who might fill any or all of these roles. Make a list. Approach them and request the type of support you want. Be as specific as possible. Rather than asking your family to "help me out," ask if they could help you by making dinner or emptying the dishwasher, for example. Let them know you are trying to start a healthier lifestyle and why their support is so important to you.

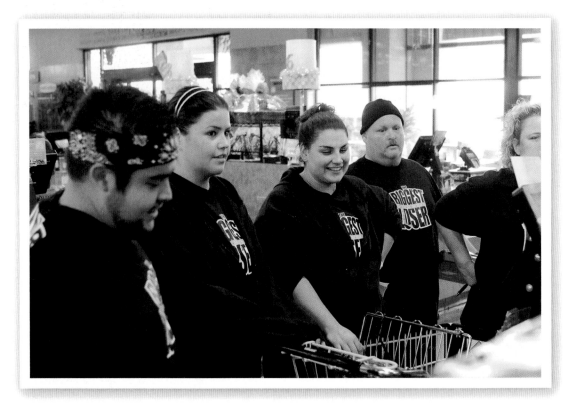

What should you do if there are no likely prospects for support in your current circle of friends? There are a variety of ways to seek out the assistance you need. You could explain the nature of your weight-loss program to your over-weight friends and ask if they'd like to join you. You might find an ally at the health club or at a dancing class. You might want to join an estab-lished support group, such as Overeaters Anony-mous, a local women's or men's support group, or a church-sponsored group. You might consider forming your own support group by advertising in your local newspaper. "Get a trainer, go to a nutritionist, go to your doctor, go to friends and family, and start telling them about your goals," says Marty Wolff, Season 3. "You will find that people around you will do nothing but help you and join in."

Adds Drea Baptiste, Season 1: "Most of the people I've met since being on the show have been so encouraging and so positive. But there are a few who say we were successful only because we had personal trainers. To them, I say, 'You have a trainer in your house too, and you don't have to pay hun-dreds of dollars for him or her. That trainer may be in the form of *The Biggest Loser Fitness* DVD or another DVD you like. All of those recordings you have in your house contain "personal trainers." Just like *The Biggest Loser* trainers at the ranch, they can stand there and tell you what to do, but it won't

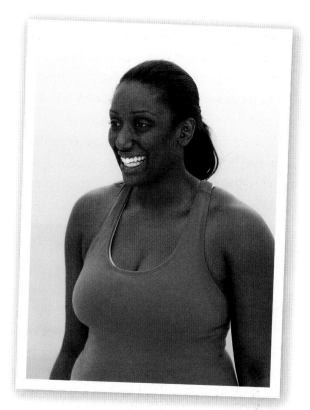

BIGGEST LOSER TOOLBOX

"If you can't find a friend who wants to be your fitness partner, try running an ad in your company's newsletter, post a bulletin at a community center—or join the Online Club. Do whatever you have to do within reason to find a partner! You both will be the better for it."

—Pete Thomas, Season 2

work until you do it. So just pop in the videotape or DVD and get to work!'"

Your support system could even be of a different ilk—books or online support groups like *The Biggest Loser* Online Club. Reading articles and books on nutrition and exercise is an excellent inducement because it increases your knowledge of fitness and helps you maintain your motivation. That's exactly what Season 2's Pete Thomas did. "Once I left the ranch, I began to research exercise and nutrition on my own, in addition to what the trainers had taught me," he says. Obviously, that strategy worked for Pete. He's maintaining an astonishing 165-pound weight loss.

As you're dropping pounds and keeping them off, the right Internet-based program can provide support and accountability and help you maintain your weight loss as effectively as a structured in-person program can, according to a 12-month University of Vermont study.

When you shop around for an online program, think about your needs: Great support from others? Delicious recipes? Advice from experts? A diet and exercise planner? Help with setting goals? One Web source to consider for support is *The Biggest Loser* Online Club at www.biggestloserclub.com, a powerful community geared toward helping you get the slender, toned, fit, and healthy body you want—for life. On the Web site you'll find menus, advice from experts and trainers, and support from real-life people who had hundreds of pounds to lose and did it—really did it! You can also meet the cast in a personal and riveting way. You'll read more about their stories and learn about their breaking points and how they turned it all around.

Remember, your relationships can help or hinder your weight loss. It's your responsibility to create an environment that leads to positive change. One final point: don't forget to show thanks and appreciation to your team! Not only will this strengthen your relationship with them, it also will reinforce their supportive behavior and make it more likely that they will continue to help you in the future.

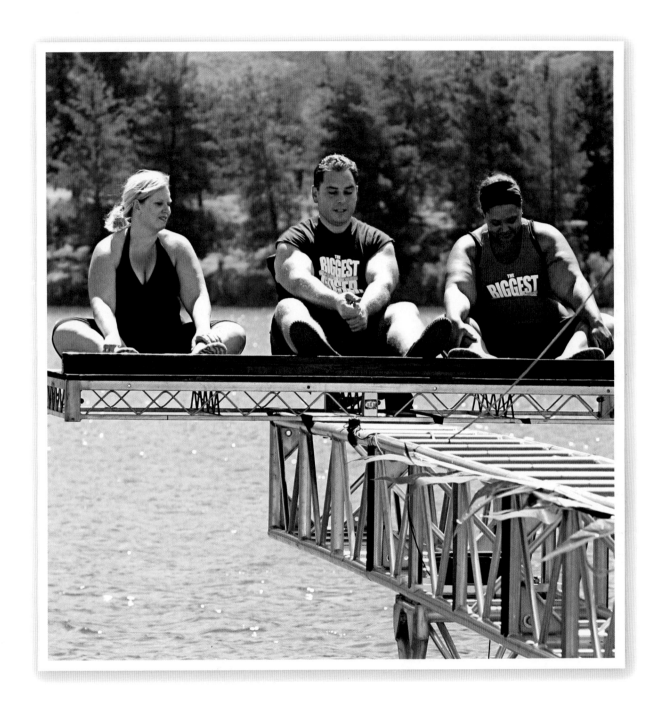

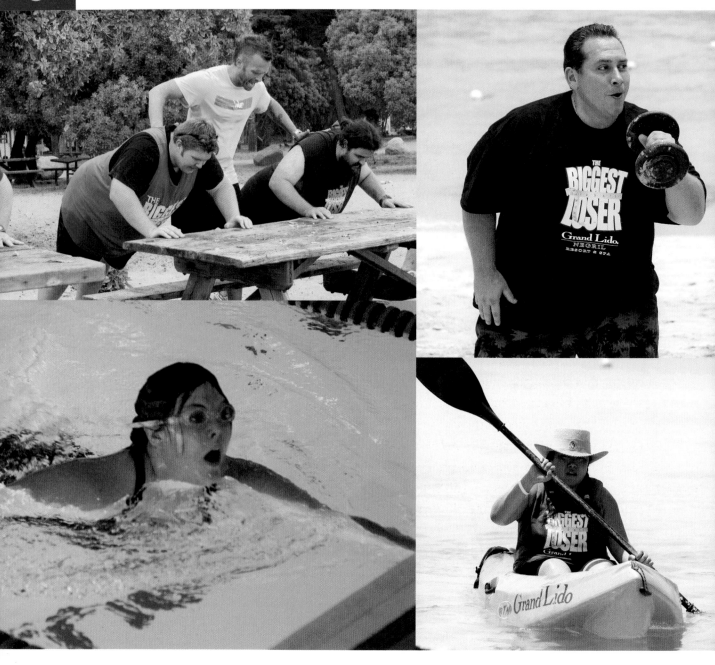

The Post-Loser Lifestyle: Living Fit

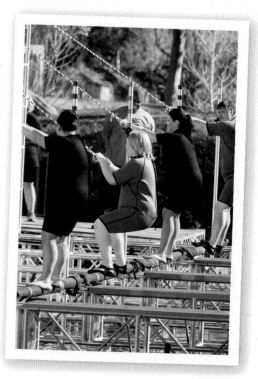

Now that you know how they lost it, you're probably wondering how the Biggest Losers keep the weight off.

"The motivation to continue—even after you've lost the weight—is one of the most difficult things about weight loss," says Michael Dansinger, MD, the leading diet and obesity researcher who helped design *The Biggest Loser* diet. "Many diet researchers are still trying to figure out what constitutes the best diet. Hardly anyone is answering the question 'How can we help people stick to the plan?' It's not human nature to force yourself to be accountable in the long term, which is why diets often succeed initially, then fail within months."

But since appearing on the show, the majority of the Biggest Losers *have* kept their weight in check, and many have

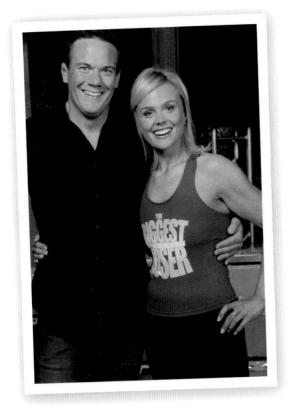

maintained their weight loss for more than a year. This is a feat that experts like Dr. Dansinger say defies the odds, particularly in our food-focused, sedentary world, where portions are large and the TV remote rules. It is very challenging to stop eating and start moving when you live in an environment that encourages this lifestyle. No wonder so many people fail at dieting.

The Biggest Losers are an exception to this rule. They keep their weight off by making permanent changes to their daily eating, exercise, and lifestyle. We're talking changes so easy to make that it's hard

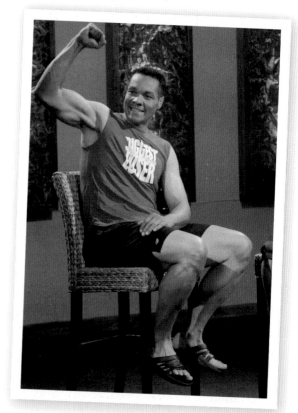

BIGGEST LOSER TOOLBOX

"Include fresh fruits and vegetables as the centerpiece of your daily food plan. Fruit juice is okay, in moderation, but it contains as many calories as a soft drink, and almost no fiber. Fresh vegetables contain a healthy amount of natural fiber and usually deliver few calories. You can load up on them and feel satisfied."

—Jackie Evans, Season 5

to believe they could make much of a difference—until you realize their cumulative effect: exiled pounds and forever-fit physiques. Here's how the Biggest Losers keep it off.

"I never thought I could . . .

**. . . wear a bikini—a dream of mine.
I love wearing it!"
—Andrea "Drea" Baptiste, Season 1**

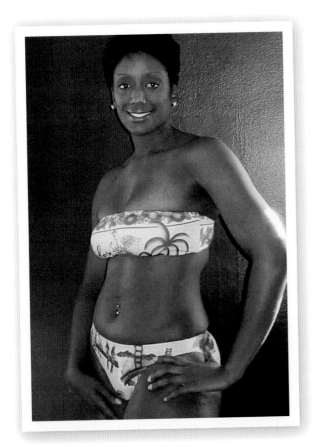

Keeping It Off, Staying Fit

It was only by changing their habits for good that Biggest Loser contestants like Matt Hoover, Suzy Preston, Pete Thomas, Andrea "Drea" Baptiste, Erik Chopin, Kelly MacFarland, and other cast members shed pounds and kept them off. "The little things that you do every day help keep you on track, like exercising, monitoring your weight, eating small meals throughout the day, and the other strategies we learned at the ranch," Kelly says. "It's not about depriving yourself or exercising like a maniac.

"Once you have positive habits you like, you wouldn't think of not doing them," she adds. "The Biggest Losers who have stayed trim just do these things and have made them a part of their lifestyle. After a while, it doesn't take such a conscious effort."

BIGGEST LOSER TOOLBOX

"Skipping meals is not a good strategy, even during maintenance. People tend to think, 'If I eat less, maybe I'll have a better week.' But we found that if we deprived ourselves too much, we didn't have as good results, so make it a habit to eat all three meals plus a snack or two each day."
—Erik Chopin, Season 3 winner

Drea Baptiste, Season 1, agrees and has gone so far as to eliminate the word "diet" from her vocabulary. "That's a negative word. When you hear it, you automatically feel resistance. The keys to keeping weight off are establishing a healthy pattern of eating—no dieting in the strict sense of the word—and staying physically active. To keep weight off, you must balance the calories you consume with the calories you burn."

What Drea advises squares with current research. Studies show that people who keep exer-

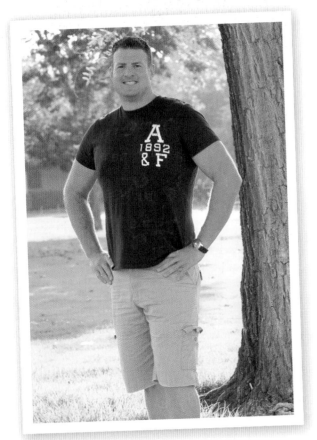

cising after losing weight maintain much, if not all, of their loss. When we weigh less, we need fewer calories to maintain our bodies, so unless we stoke up the exercise, we won't have as much flexibility with food intake.

Season 3 Biggest Loser Erik Chopin says he maintains his loss by doing an hour of cardio five or six times a week and by consuming about 2,000 quality calories a day, except for 1 day a week when he treats himself to a dessert. Because Erik's approach to maintenance is reasonable and achievable, he's been able to stay at a healthy weight.

"I never thought I could . . .

. . . ditch the maternity pants I had to wear because I was so fat. I used to have to buy them because I was so big in the middle. I'm so happy that I've been able to burn those!"
—Brittany Aberle, Season 5

Pete Thomas, Season 2, says he uses three strategies—all learned during his time at the ranch—to keep 165 pounds off: calorie control; consistent, challenging exercise; and ongoing support. Once he and his wife, Pam, started monitoring calories, for example, they realized that in one date night alone—dinner and a movie—they were packing away more than 3 days' worth of calories. "It's not just a matter of cutting back or cutting out certain foods," Pete says. "It's really about figuring out how much fuel your body needs and sticking with an exercise program that continually challenges you."

Pete's current routine includes 1 hour of full-body strength training on Mondays, Wednesdays, and Fridays and 1 hour of cardio on Tuesdays, Thursdays, and sometimes Saturdays. His favorite forms of cardio include the treadmill, the stair-climber, basketball, and spinning.

Here's more incredibly powerful news about

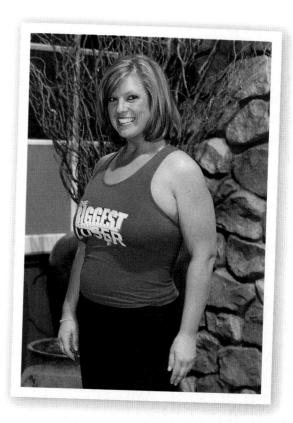

maintenance: It gets easier with time. That's the conclusion of the National Weight Control Registry—a database of thousands of people who have shed an average of 66 pounds and kept it off for an average of more than 5 years. If you can maintain your new weight for 2 years, you have a greater likelihood of keeping it off for 2 more years. And if you keep it off for 5 years, you have even greater odds of maintaining your weight loss. The longer you stay fit and trim, the more your odds of regaining weight are reduced. (For more maintenance

BIGGEST LOSER TOOLBOX

"Get rid of your fat clothes. You never want to go back there! Give away or donate all the clothes that are too big for you. Reward yourself with clothes that perfectly fit your new, trim figure."

—Julie Hadden, Season 4 runner-up

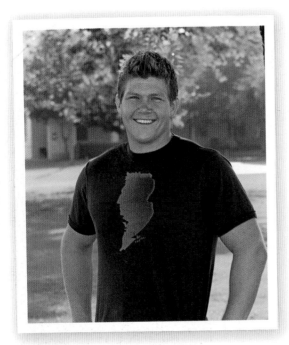

tools, check out other strategies in the Biggest Loser toolboxes throughout this chapter.)

Pay Attention to Hunger Management

Managing hunger is a little-known secret to losing pounds and keeping them from coming back, but it's one that all the Biggest Losers know about and use. Your body is equipped with two signals that tell you when to eat and how much to eat. The "when" signal is hunger; the "how much" signal is satiety (the feeling of fullness). They work in tandem with one another. The body sends a hunger signal—in the form of hunger pangs, weakness, or diminished attention span. Eating a meal relieves these feelings. People who eat in response to physical hunger tend to be in pretty good shape. Others, who are out of touch with these sensations, are highly responsive to environmental and emotional cues. They eat because an emotion needs to be calmed, because the clock says it's time, or because they are tempted by delicious food. People who eat for reasons other than true physical hunger may struggle with their weight.

About 20 minutes into the meal, the body sends satiety signals. You feel full and don't want to eat any more. If you gulp down your food in less than 20 minutes, you're likely to keep eating because your satiety signal hasn't yet been sent. "Stretching

BIGGEST LOSER TOOLBOX

"Stay on top of your weight at least weekly. You don't have to stay at your exact goal weight all the time, but aim to keep within a few pounds of it. If you go up a couple of pounds, you need to cut back a bit on the eating, or increase your exercise, before 5 pounds becomes 15 or 50. Set a limit for regaining weight—like 5 pounds. If you reach it, make a quick course correction. Switch from weight maintenance back to weight loss."

—Kelly MacFarland, Season 1

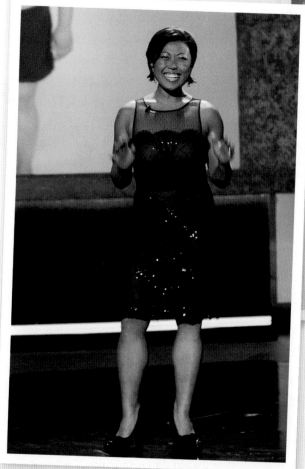

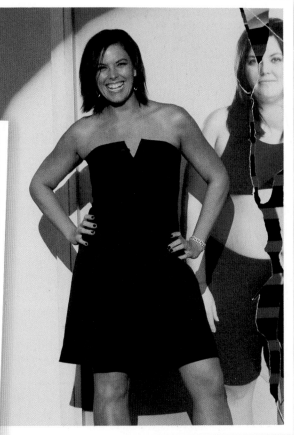

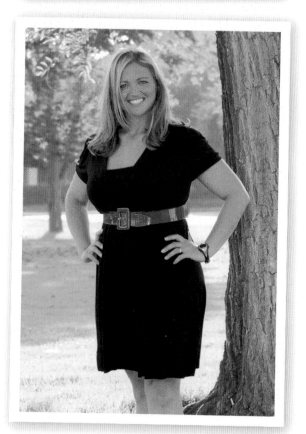

out your meal for at least 20 minutes helps you eat just the right amount," advises Matt Hoover, Season 2's winner. "If you eat when you're hungry and stop when you're full, you'll have an easier time keeping your weight in check." You'll also have the added benefit of feeling satisfied yet energetic after a meal, instead of overly full and sluggish.

Healthy people pay attention to these signals. "They are willing to adjust their food choices in such a way that they are working with their body and not against it," adds Greg Hottinger, *The Biggest Loser* Online Club expert. "They pay close attention to their hunger and fullness signals and notice that they feel better when they stay balanced, not too hungry and not too full."

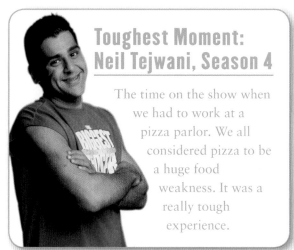

"I never thought I could . . .

. . . face the world without fear. I was always afraid of how I'd be judged, so I never stepped out and did anything that would help me realize my dreams."
—Isabeau Miller, Season 4

Exercise Mind over Platter

Show psychologist Alexa Altman is often asked what psychological factors help people maintain their weight loss. From her clinical experience and work with contestants, Altman believes that successful losers have certain psychological similarities.

First, goal setting does not stop when you reach maintenance. (Remember Pete Thomas's advice about creating two sets of goals—one for losing and one for maintaining?) Successful Biggest

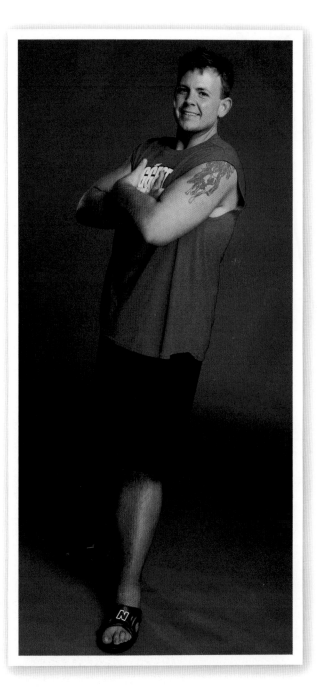

BIGGEST LOSER TOOLBOX

"Keep putting yourself first. My weight issue was an indirect result of my devotion to my students. I focused so much on them that 'me' time was often takeout and TV. I now make myself and my well-being a priority. I'm finally putting my health first, and that feels fabulous."
—Hollie Self, Season 4 finalist

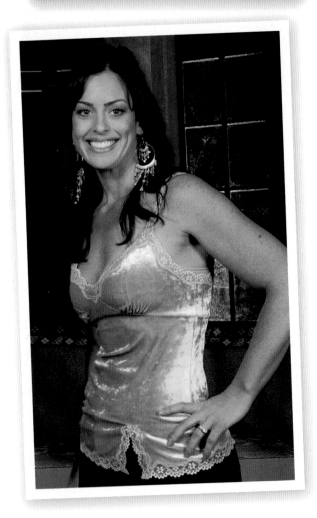

Losers never lose sight of such goals. In fact, they review their goals daily.

Second, they think in shades of gray. "Most of us think in black and white, and we divide our world into nice and neat categories," Altman explains. "'I am good' or 'I am bad.' This is a setup for disaster, however, in that one small mistake becomes a failure. Successful Biggest Losers don't interpret a small slipup as a failure; they get back on the horse right away."

Third, successful Biggest Losers utilize resources, which include anything that contributes to your success and well-being. "If I told you that you were about to go on the longest journey of a lifetime, you would want to pack your bag and make sure you had enough clothes, water, food, and so forth," says Altman. "It's necessary to establish what resources will be needed for success. Do you need a nutritionist, fitness instructor, food journal, online support group, set of recipes, or psychotherapist, for example?"

Finally, successful Biggest Losers identify problems early and figure out what is getting in their way. "Is it emotional eating, depression,

"I never thought I could . . .
. . . run! When I work out now, I can run for almost an hour. It's totally amazing."
—Jackie Evans, Season 5

anxiety, recent losses, work stress?" Altman says. "Do you want to address the big roadblock right in the middle of your path or continue to walk over and around it? What do you gain by continuing to avoid what might be sabotaging your success? This is an opportunity to make real life changes." (The flag system described in Chapter 5 is an excellent tool to help you pinpoint slipups before they become problems.)

If you notice there is an area that needs further attention, don't beat yourself up about it, Altman emphasizes. "This is an opportunity for you to expand and enrich your life," she says.

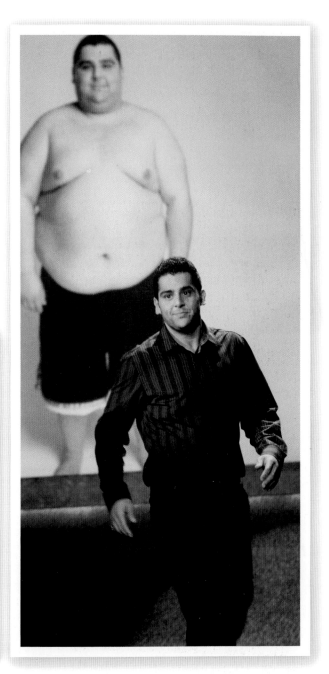

BIGGEST LOSER TOOLBOX

"Weight maintenance starts when you decide to lose weight. I had lost 100 pounds earlier in my life. What was different about *The Biggest Loser* was that I had to step out in front of people and admit, hey, something's wrong with me. Before, I tried to do it all on my own, behind closed doors, where no one could see me. But you don't have to be on *The Biggest Loser* to go public. Announce to people that you have a problem with your weight, that you want to do something about it, and that after you lose it, you want to keep it off. Declare it in the beginning and you'll keep it off in the end."

—Marty Wolff, Season 3

"Examine your strengths, too. When you notice an area of particular strength, take a moment to assess how this has helped you in attaining a healthier mind and body. It is helpful to acknowledge what you are doing well. When you notice an area of particular weakness, notice how this may be limiting your success or contributing to unhealthy behaviors. Think about how you can begin to build or strengthen one of these areas."

Be Fit as a Family

The Biggest Losers agree that when they change, a change in family lifestyle has to follow to make it stick for a lifetime. Family life can be a huge factor in a child's health, as well as your own. Children learn primarily by their parents' example. If your eating and exercise habits are poor, your children's will probably be unhealthy, too. But if you can

The Biggest Loser Online Club Profile: **Mary Averill**

Starting weight: 260 • Current weight: 158 • Goal weight: 160

Mary was always worried about the effect of her excess weight on her health. But once she joined *The Biggest Loser* Online Club, she gained the tools she needed to see real weight-loss success. The consistent weight loss she experienced from week to week kept her motivated to continue.

"Exercise is one reason I am maintaining my goal of a size 10—which beats a size 24 anytime," she says. "I recently ran a 5K race and have three more planned. I never would have believed any of this would have been possible a year ago."

Mary recommends using a pedometer. "It gives you an idea of how much you're moving. Try to take more steps every day. You will actually begin to like it. You will get to a point where you miss it when you don't get a chance to work out. As your fitness level improves you will be *amazed* at what you can do."

Mary's biggest challenges on the road to reaching her goal were implementing her *Biggest Loser* Online Club food plan while also feeding her family. "I had to focus on me this time. Luckily, my kids are teenagers and old enough to fend for themselves for a while. I just kept the kitchen well stocked and they were able to let me concentrate on cooking for me."

Change your life today! Log on to www.biggestloserclub.com and get started.

establish yourself as a positive role model, your kids have a better chance of adopting lifelong healthful habits at an early age and avoiding falling victim to childhood obesity, which has become an epidemic in the United States.

The challenge, though, is to make family fitness a habit. These days, we're all so busy that commitments—even family commitments—can get in the way of a consistent fitness program. When you have kids, it's often difficult to find time for exercise.

In his post-loser life, Season 2's Pete Thomas, who does not yet have kids, is passionate about helping children become more active and fit. He works with an organization that teaches children and their families to take ownership of their health through physical activity and balanced eating. The organization delivers exercise equipment to kids, shows them how to use it, and teaches them about nutrition and healthy eating habits.

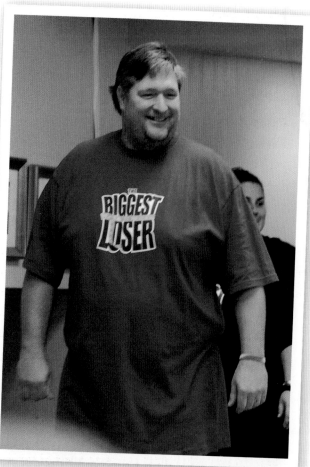

> "I never thought I could . . .
> . . . do anything athletic. I couldn't walk up stairs before, and now I do triathlons!"
> —Kelly MacFarland, Season 1

Best Moment: Isabeau Miller, Season 4

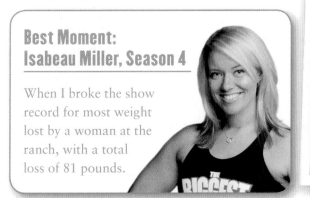

When I broke the show record for most weight lost by a woman at the ranch, with a total loss of 81 pounds.

"It's one of many ways to promote family fitness," Pete says. "I believe the reason so many children are overweight has to do with the parents. Some parents are just feeding their kids to death. But you don't have to express your love to your child through food."

Pete and his wife, Pam, have made many changes in their lifestyle, including the way they vacation. "We used to plan our vacations around

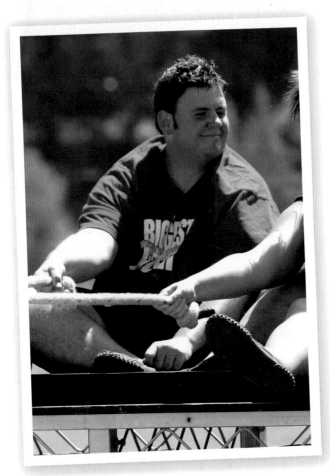

eating, like going to Chicago so we could go to restaurants," says Pam, who dropped 70 pounds while Pete was losing his weight. "Now our vacations are activity-related." During their last trip to Chicago, they biked along the city's lakeshore and walked around the museums. During a California trip, they went hiking—experiences they loved. "Any time you go through a struggle and triumph together, it makes you stronger," Pete says. "For us, that struggle was losing weight."

Other Biggest Losers share Pete's passion for helping families become more fit by exercising together. David Griffin, Season 4, believes that family fitness can—and should—be fun. "Keep a healthy balance between play and exercise," he advises. "Incorporate fun fitness activities such as bike riding, horseback riding, or outdoor games that give you a great workout, such as tag, softball, volleyball, or tossing a Frisbee. These days, most health clubs are family friendly and promote activities family members can do together. The minute kids think it's a grind, you've lost them."

One of the biggest challenges is to encourage healthy eating in the home. Mark Kruger, Season 5, says you have to make it hard to eat unhealthy foods. He came up with a strategy to nip his ice cream habit in the bud—a habit that also helps his family. "Instead of buying a gallon of ice cream and keeping it in the freezer, we take our family to the ice cream store and indulge in a scoop rather than a bowl. If we absolutely have to have ice cream around, we buy the reduced-fat or sugar-free versions of our favorite ice cream and enjoy those instead."

At Roger Shultz's house, healthy snacks are left in plain view. "We keep a bowl of fresh fruit on the counter. It's easy for the kids to reach for those. Because it's convenient, it helps keep them away from unhealthy choices," says the Season 5 contestant.

Adds Season 2's Andrea Overstreet, "Let children be a part of the meal planning. If they select it, they are more likely to eat it."

Another strategy is to limit television time. It cuts down on the amount of time kids may spend snacking on no-nutrient junk foods and adds time for play and physical activity. At an American Heart Association meeting, a California researcher reported that children who watch too much TV may actually be more likely to develop heart disease later in life. The cholesterol levels and viewing

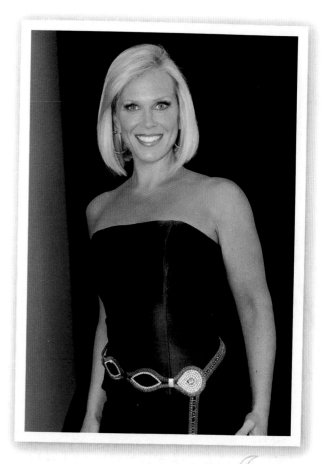

BIGGEST LOSER TOOLBOX

"Reward yourself for sticking to healthy habits with things unrelated to food, such as a massage, *The Biggest Loser* DVD, new workout clothes, a haircut, or a new outfit. Your reward should be a true treat—something you don't often do for yourself."
—Pam Smith, Season 3

habits of 1,066 children and adolescents ages 2 to 20 were examined, and the results showed that watching 2 or more hours of TV daily is the strongest risk factor for elevated cholesterol in that age group. Television isn't the bad guy, though. It's what kids do when they're watching it. Children tend to spend time eating and being sedentary in front of the TV rather than going outside to play. "It might sound like tough love," says David

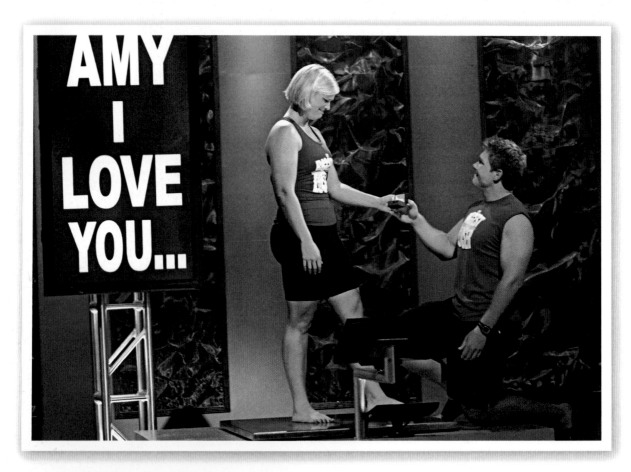

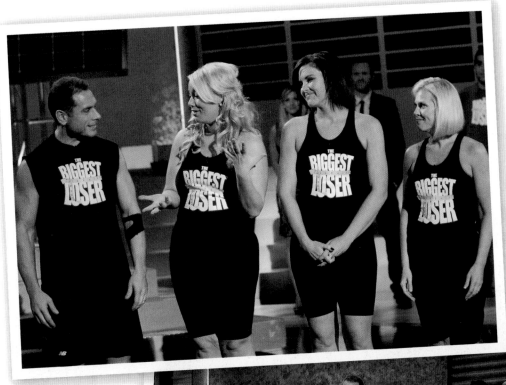

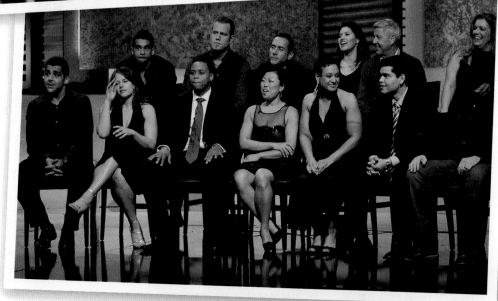

Griffin, Season 4, "but turning off the TV on occasion is a loving gift to your kids in terms of their health and quality family time."

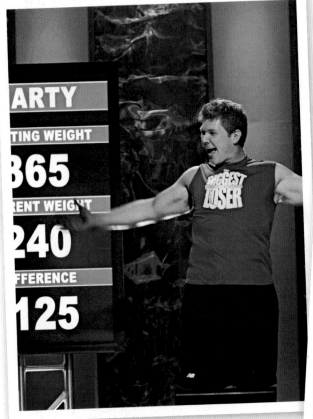

Start Thinking like a Fit Person

One of the main reasons fit, healthy people stay that way isn't simply because of good genes. They think about food and exercise in ways that keep pounds off. The good news is that anyone can develop the same mind-set—and lose weight and keep it off. Greg Hottinger, *The Biggest Loser* Online Club expert, has developed these tips to help you think fit—and be fit.

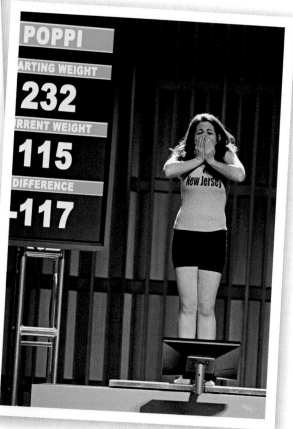

- **Cultivate an attitude of fun.** Fit, healthy people enjoy activity for the sake of the activity. It could be a night of dancing, a hard-fought tennis match, or a hike with a good friend. But the value is intrinsic. The fact that the activity also happens to be "good for you" is secondary. Find an activity that you would choose to do without knowing it's good for you, or something you would miss doing if you no longer could.

- **Enjoy active chores and tasks.** Fit, healthy people do not view daily activities and chores as taxing, and they revel in being able to do these things easily. Instead of avoiding mowing the lawn, chopping wood, or raking leaves, fit people look at chores as an opportunity to lift, squat, walk, lunge, twist, pull—you get the picture! Why wait to be at a gym? To adopt a similar mind-set, pick an errand or task around the house that could be a "mini-workout." As you do it, think about the similarities to some of the movements you do at the gym. What skills and strengths that you've built at the gym are you now using in everyday life?

- **Make activity a positive addiction.** Fit, healthy people "hook" into exercise by signing up for classes, playing in sports leagues, exercising with partners, or joining clubs based on activities like hiking. Take a look at your local paper and look for upcoming events, group meetings,

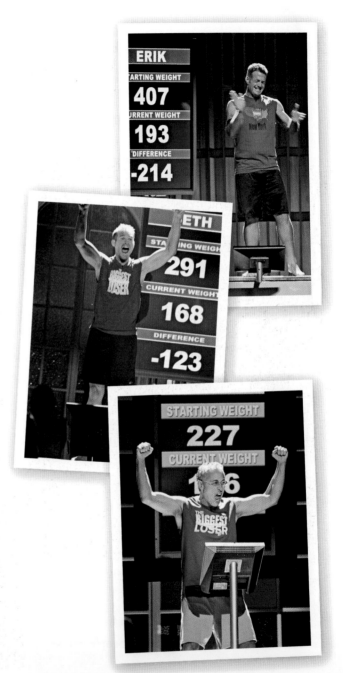

trips, or classes. Commit to signing up and participating in one event by the end of the month.

- **Don't be fooled by portion traps.** Fit, healthy people do not succumb to the "all you can eat," "supersize," or "2 for the price of 1" traps around food. They know that bigger portions lead to eating more. So they either don't buy excess food or they aren't afraid to throw it away if they do. Try this: The next time you buy food away from home, think about getting what you actually need versus getting the most for your money. Leave food on your plate and say to yourself, "I'd rather throw this food away than wear it."

- **Don't give in to second helpings.** Fit, healthy people know that the meal sitting before them is not their Last Supper. In fact, they've noticed that when they don't overeat at this meal, they enjoy their next meal even more. They consider food part of the celebration, not the reason for it. The next time you feel tempted to have that second plate of food, remind yourself that you'll be eating again in just a few hours. Take a couple of deep breaths and focus on the sensations in your body. If you still feel a strong desire to eat more, give yourself three more bites and then push the food away.

- **Make the connection between being fit and the rest of your life.** Fit, healthy people can see the connection between being fit and doing other things they find enjoyable. Traveling, gardening, having sex, going to the theater, and shopping are just a few of the things that are enhanced by fitness. Here's something to try: Use a backpack to carry weight equal to what you have lost. Wear it while you go shopping, walk in the park, or do some other fun activity this weekend. Then, while still in the midst of your fun, take it off. Savor the difference and know that there is more to come!

There is a natural ecstasy that comes with having a fit body—and you can experience it! Decide today that you'll employ these *Biggest Loser* strategies—and that you're no longer going to live in an overburdened body, but instead in one that moves, breathes, and lives in healthy liberty.

As you begin to commit to these strategies, try not to look at diet, exercise, and maintenance as chores to be endured, but as welcome challenges that will take your body to new levels of health and fitness. Just think about what you'll gain once you reach your destination: a leaner, fitter figure; more energy and greater stamina; sounder sleep; improved general health; greater confidence; less stress and anxiety; a better outlook on life; and more.

Who wouldn't want all that?

Now . . . go for it!

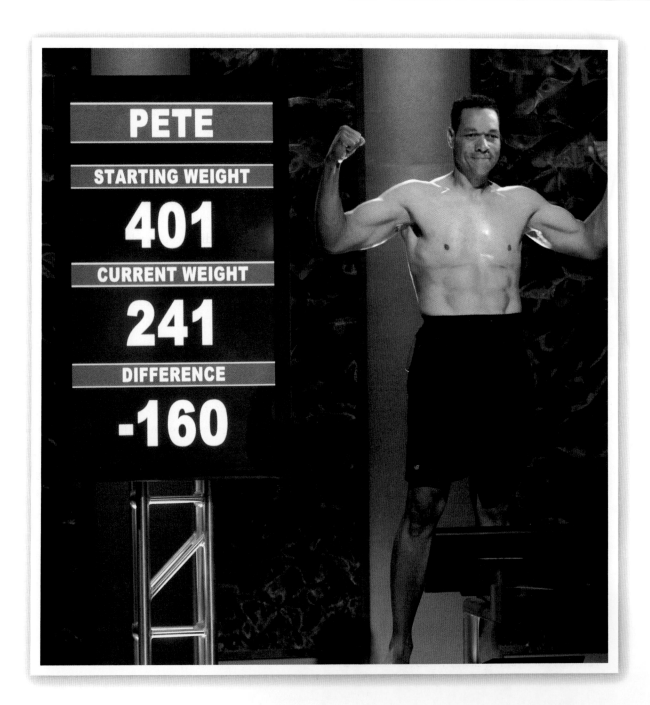

PETE

STARTING WEIGHT
401

CURRENT WEIGHT
241

DIFFERENCE
-160

References

Elfhag, K., and S. Rossner. 2005. "Who succeeds in maintaining weight loss? A conceptual review of factors associated with weight loss maintenance and weight regain." *Obesity Reviews* 6: 67–85.

Gorin, A. A., et al. 2004. "Medical triggers are associated with better short- and long-term weight loss outcomes." *Preventive Medicine* 39(3): 612–616.

Klem, M. L., et al. 1997. "A descriptive study of individuals successful at long-term maintenance of substantial weight loss." *American Journal of Clinical Nutrition* 66: 239–246.

———. 2000. "Does weight loss maintenance become easier over time?" *Obesity Research* 8: 438–444.

Lichtman, S. W., et al. 1992. "Discrepancy between self-reported and actual calorie intake and exercise in obese subjects." *The New England Journal of Medicine* 327: 1893–1898.

Wallace, J. P., et al. 1995. "Twelve month adherence of adults who joined a fitness program with a spouse vs without a spouse." *Journal of Sports Medicine and Physical Fitness* 35: 206–213.

Wing, R. R., et al. 2006. "A self-regulation program for maintenance of weight loss." *The New England Journal of Medicine* 355: 1563–1571.

Resources

For even greater inspiration as you begin your own Biggest Loser journey, check out these tools and resources, available online from *The Biggest Loser* Online Club Web site at www.biggestloserclub.com or through the NBC Store at www.nbcstore.com.

Books

The Biggest Loser, the first book, provides fitness advice from trainers Bob Harper and Jillian Michaels, eating plans from the show's medical experts, and tips and weight-loss stories from contestants.

The Biggest Loser Cookbook features delicious recipes from Chef Devin Alexander and the Biggest Loser experts and cast members. With more than 125 guilt-free, flavorful recipes, this cookbook shows that healthy eating and successful weight loss doesn't mean giving up your favorite foods.

The Biggest Loser Calorie Counter provides a listing of the caloric totals for approximately 7,500 common foods. The book includes advice for dining out in common restaurants, Biggest Loser contestant and trainer tips, suggestions for substitutions, and Top 20 lists (20 Low-Calorie Desserts to Die For, 20 Low-Cal Treats to Cure Your Worst Cravings, 20 Best Options for Evening Snacks)

The Biggest Loser Fitness Program showcases the personalized fitness program used by Biggest Loser contestants to dramatically transform their bodies and lives! In addition, this book offers sensible and real-life eating advice from the show's nutrition experts, dozens of tips and tricks for getting started from the show's trainers and contestants, inspiring and motivating contestant testimonials, including before-and-after photos, clear, how-to photographs for each workout move, and modifications for beginners and advanced readers alike.

DVDs

Biggest Loser: The Workout, Volume One, offers six different fun workout routines adapted from the show and features trainer Bob Harper as well as support from the cast.

Biggest Loser: The Workout, Volume Two, includes workouts specifically designed for men and women and a customized option allowing you to mix and match your workout according to your current fitness level. Since weight loss is also about nutrition and lifestyle, there is both an inspirational segment and a nutritional cooking segment.

The Biggest Loser Workout: Cardio Max provides a 6-week program that begins with Level 1 and, as you progress, adds on Levels 2 and 3. In no time, those extra pounds will disappear and your body will transform before your eyes.

The Biggest Loser Workout: Power Sculpt features the sculpting techniques of your favorite power-training trio: Bob, Kim, and Jillian. Just like on NBC's hit show, you will increase strength, blast maximum calories, and transform your body in a minimum of time. For best results, follow the 6-week program that begins with Level 1 and, as you progress, adds on Levels 2 and 3. Before you know it, you will chisel away unwanted pounds to reveal a leaner, stronger you!

The Biggest Loser Online Club at www.biggestloserclub.com offers detailed meal and fitness plans, access to experts and past contestants from the show, support groups, and daily tips. It has more than 75,000 members and is now the third-most-popular health and lifestyle subscription site online.

The Biggest Loser Magazine is the newest addition to all the great Biggest Loser resources. It is loaded with diet and fitness tips, recipes, and up-close-and-personal stories with the Biggest Loser cast. Pick up an issue wherever magazines are sold.

Acknowledgments

There are more Biggest Losers than ever before, not only after five seasons of this inspiring show but also from the many *Biggest Loser* Online Club members who are losing weight right at home. My thanks go out to all of these people, first of all, for honestly and graciously sharing their stories, successes, and strategies so that millions of readers can be Biggest Losers for life, and to the nutrition and medical experts whom you don't usually see on television but are doing life-saving work behind the scenes and through *The Biggest Loser* Online Club.

We had a very ambitious deadline for producing this book and in true team spirit, everyone pulled together to make it happen. My thanks go to our editor, Julie Will, for her expert guidance, astute editing, and creative insight; interior designer Chris Gaugler, for a book design so vivid that it makes you feel like you're on the ranch; cover designer Chris Rhoads, for designing another beautiful cover; project editor Nancy N. Bailey, for her organization and skill; copy editors Nancy Elgin and Beth Bazar, for their talented work; and to the publisher of Rodale Books, Liz Perl, and Executive Editor Nancy Hancock, for their dedication to this series.

Chad Bennett, once again, was the superb point person for all things Biggest Loser who coordinated this entire project, making sure that nothing was left undone. Thank you also to Mark Koops, managing director, cohead of Domestic Television of Reveille, and Cindy Chang and Kim Niemi at NBC Universal for their commitment to taking *The Biggest Loser* message, program, and philosophy worldwide.

Maggie Greenwood-Robinson, PhD
Dallas, Texas

Index

Underscored page references indicate boxed text. **Boldface** references indicate photographs.

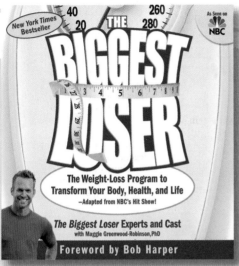
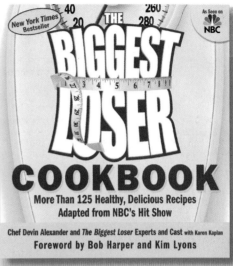
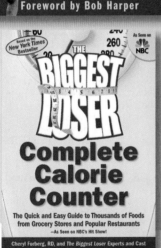
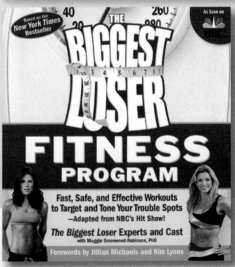
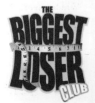

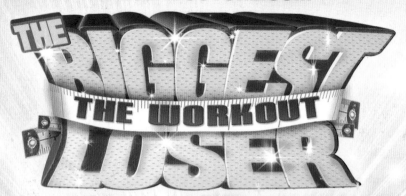
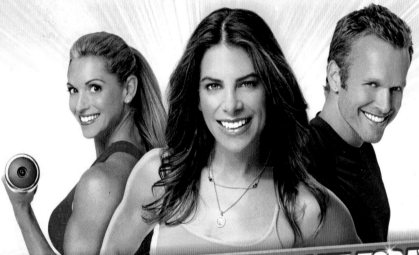
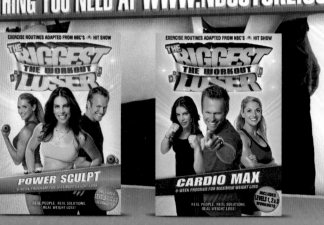